To all those pulmonary rehabilitation health care providers who,
without fanfare and often without sufficient reimbursement,
out of dedication, continue to provide this much-needed service.

third edition

Guidelines for Pulmonary Rehabilitation Programs

American
and I
Promotir

Books are to be returned on or before
the last date below.

7 – DAY
LOAN

ar

Human Kinetics

Library of Congress Cataloging-in-Publication Data

American Association of Cardiovascular & Pulmonary Rehabilitation.
  Guidelines for pulmonary rehabilitation programs / American Association of
Cardiovascular & Pulmonary Rehabilitation.-- 3rd ed.
     p. ; cm.
  Includes bibliographical references and index.
  ISBN 0-7360-5573-8 (soft cover)
  1. Lungs--Diseases, Obstructive--Patients--Rehabilitation--Standards. 2.
Lungs--Diseases--Patients--Rehabilitation--Standards. 3. Respiratory therapy--
Standards.
  [DNLM: 1. Lung Diseases, Obstructive--rehabilitation. 2. Needs Assessment.
3. Patient Education. 4. Rehabilitation--standards. 5. Treatment Outcome. WF
600 A5117g 2005] I. Title.
  RC776.O3A64 2005
  616.2'403--dc22

                                          2004010721

ISBN: 0-7360-5573-8

The Web addresses cited in this text were current as of June 18, 2004, unless otherwise noted.

Acquisitions Editor: Loarn D. Robertson, PhD; **Managing Editor:** Amanda S. Ewing; **Assistant Editor:** Bethany J. Bentley; **Copyeditor:** Patsy Fortney; **Proofreader:** Sarah Wiseman; **Indexer:** Dan Connolly; **Permission Manager:** Dalene Reeder; **Graphic Designer:** Nancy Rasmus; **Graphic Artist:** Denise Lowry; **Photo Manager:** Kareema McLendon; **Cover Designer:** Keith Blomberg; **Photographer (interior):** Kelly J. Huff, unless otherwise noted; **Art Manager:** Kelly Hendren; **Illustrator:** Kelly Hendren; **Printer:** United Graphics

We thank the Duke Center for Living, Duke University Medical Center in Durham, North Carolina, for assistance in providing the location for the photo shoot for this book.

Printed in the United States of America   10 9 8 7 6 5 4 3 2

Human Kinetics
Web site: www.HumanKinetics.com

United States: Human Kinetics, P.O. Box 5076, Champaign, IL 61825-5076
800-747-4457
e-mail: humank@hkusa.com

Canada: Human Kinetics, 475 Devonshire Road, Unit 100, Windsor, ON N8Y 2L5
800-465-7301 (in Canada only)
e-mail: orders@hkcanada.com

Europe: Human Kinetics, 107 Bradford Road, Stanningley
Leeds LS28 6AT, United Kingdom
+44 (0) 113 255 5665
e-mail: hk@hkeurope.com

Australia: Human Kinetics, 57A Price Avenue, Lower Mitcham, South Australia 5062
08 8277 1555
e-mail: liaw@hkaustralia.com

New Zealand: Human Kinetics, Division of Sports Distributors NZ Ltd.
P.O. Box 300 226 Albany, North Shore City, Auckland
0064 9 448 1207
e-mail: info@humankinetics.co.nz

contents

preface

The goal of the third edition of the American Association of Cardiovascular and Pulmonary Rehabilitation's (AACVPR's) *Guidelines for Pulmonary Rehabilitation Programs* is to provide a scientific and practical framework for the optimal delivery of pulmonary rehabilitation to people with symptomatic respiratory disease. This third edition outlines the essentials required to design and implement (or update) a program. It also offers practitioners an understanding of the theory of pulmonary rehabilitation, as well as the close association between the AACVPR program credentialing process and these guidelines. The guidelines are intended for all health care providers involved in pulmonary rehabilitation. They are written to address outpatient pulmonary rehabilitation services, but they may be used in an inpatient setting with appropriate modification. This edition will address the following:

- The essential components of pulmonary rehabilitation, including assessment, patient education and training, therapeutic and supervised exercise, psychosocial intervention, long-term adherence, outcomes, and prevention
- The integration of long-term adherence, maintenance of gains, and prevention into pulmonary rehabilitation
- Earlier screening and detection of lung disease "test your lungs know your numbers" and ways to make pulmonary rehabilitation more accessible to patients

- Patient selection criteria for any patient with chronic respiratory disease who remains symptomatic despite maximum medical therapy
- The need for rehabilitation services tailored to the patient's individual needs
- The importance of outcome documentation

These guidelines are intended for the following groups:

- Health professionals (interdisciplinary team members) developing and updating pulmonary rehabilitation services
- Physicians and other allied health care professionals referring patients for pulmonary rehabilitation
- Patients and significant others interested in knowing what pulmonary rehabilitation services should consist of prior to selecting a service
- Third-party payers evaluating pulmonary rehabilitation services
- Educators training health care professionals (e.g., respiratory therapists, nurses, pulmonary fellows, physicians, physical therapists, occupational therapists, and exercise physiologists) in pulmonary rehabilitation
- Individuals involved in educating the media and public about pulmonary rehabilitation
- Facilities applying for AACVPR pulmonary rehabilitation program certification

acknowledgments

As co-chairs of the writing committee of the AACVPR's *Guidelines for Pulmonary Rehabilitation, third edition,* we would like to individually thank the members of the writing committee for their efforts and dedication in producing this document. Each chapter was assigned a captain whose job was to revise the existing chapter from the second edition. Intense discussion and deliberation involving the entire committee on each new chapter followed. Despite heated discussions, we are still friends.

In particular, we would like to acknowledge the following members. Lana Hilling and GeriLynn Connors, who as co-chairs of the first and second editions, brought their invaluable experience to the table. They also were instrumental in revising chapter 1, *Overview of Pulmonary Rehabilitation,* and chapter 8, *Program Management.* Jon Raskin brought his considerable experience in pulmonary rehabilitation to the committee and helped in all chapters, especially in chapter 8, *Program Management.* Linda Nici did an admirable job rewriting chapter 2, *Selection and Assessment of the Pulmonary Rehabilitation Candidate.* Bonnie Fahy, as expected, did a superb job with chapter 3, *Patient Education and Skills Training.* Neil MacIntyre brought his in-depth knowledge and experience in exercise testing and training to revise chapter 4, *Exercise Assessment and Training.* Dr. MacIntyre was also very helpful in our committee's formulating specific recommendations in areas of assessment, exercise training, education, and psychosocial support. Jane Reardon was responsible for the initial draft of chapter 5, *Psychosocial Assessment and Intervention,* which was so well written it needed only minor revisions. Gretchen Peske captained chapter 6, *Outcome Assessment,* which was essentially completely revised from the second edition. Finally, Carly Rochester wrote chapter 7, *Disease-Specific Approaches in Pulmonary Rehabilitation.* This chapter, in our opinion, is the best scholarly review of the approaches to the pulmonary rehabilitation of the non-COPD patient existing in the medical literature.

Rebecca Crouch and **Richard ZuWallack**

Guidelines for Pulmonary Rehabilitation Programs, Third Edition Working Group:

Co-chairs:

Rebecca H. Crouch, PT, MS, FAACVPR

Richard ZuWallack, MD, FAACVPR

Gerilynn Connors, BS, RRT, FAACVPR

Bonnie Fahy, RN, MN, FAACVPR

Lana Hilling, RCP, RRT, FAACVPR

Neil MacIntyre, MD, FAACVPR

Linda Nici, MD

Gretchen Peske, RN, MSN, FAACVPR

Jonathan Raskin, MD

Jane Reardon, RN, MSN, CS, FAACVPR

Carolyn Rochester, MD

Joanne Smith, PhD

We would also like to sincerely thank Dr. Brian Carlin for his insightful input into all of the chapters.

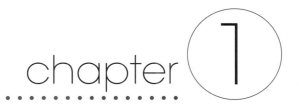
Overview of Pulmonary Rehabilitation

Today pulmonary rehabilitation is recognized as an integral component of the standard quality medical therapy for patients with chronic respiratory disease.[1,2,3] Pulmonary rehabilitation has evolved over the past 50 years in response to the increasing number of patients with chronic respiratory diseases. Its purpose is to alleviate patients' symptoms, optimize their daily function, and improve their disability from chronic respiratory disease. The strategies, therapeutic interventions, and disease management principles used in comprehensive pulmonary rehabilitation have been well established.[4,5,6] Its documented benefits are substantial and include decreased symptoms, improved quality of life, increased exercise tolerance, greater independence in activities of daily living (ADLs), and decreased use of medical resources.[4,7,8]

Despite the unequivocally positive scientific literature backing its use, the implementation of pulmonary rehabilitation still faces challenges. These include remaining skepticism from some elements of the medical community and lack of enthusiasm from some physicians. This at times leads to inadequate transfer of information on pulmonary rehabilitation to the patient, insufficient numbers of referrals, and delays in referrals. Additional challenges include inadequate program availability in some regions of the country and—at the time of this writing—the lack of a national policy to provide fair and adequate funding for these needed services.

The traditional focus of pulmonary rehabilitation has been on patients with chronic obstructive pulmonary disease (COPD). Pulmonary rehabilitation will also benefit people with other chronic respiratory conditions who remain symptomatic or have reductions in functional status following standard medical therapy. These include patients with asthma, cystic fibrosis, interstitial lung disease, obesity-related respiratory disorders, pulmonary hypertension, neuromuscular disorders, alpha-1 antitrypsin deficiency, lung volume reduction surgery for emphysema, lung transplantation, lung cancer, thoracic and upper abdominal surgery, and mechanical ventilation, as well as some pediatric patients with respiratory disease and selected patients with coexisting respiratory and cardiac disease (see chapter 7).

This chapter provides a brief preview of subsequent chapters and covers a variety of topics in comprehensive pulmonary rehabilitation: its definition and scope, the burden of chronic respiratory disease on our society, a historical overview, the components of pulmonary rehabilitation, the need to focus on prevention of respiratory disease, examples of patient and program goals, and a suggested code of ethics.

Each of these topics is critical to understanding pulmonary rehabilitation and to developing or updating successful services. An understanding of the definition and scope of pulmonary rehabilitation will set the foundation for pulmonary rehabilitation services. Reviewing the epidemiological data of lung disease will underscore the need for this intervention in patients with chronic respiratory disease. Knowledge of the historical roots and the more recent scientific evidence supporting pulmonary rehabilitation will provide an appreciation of the strong footing underlying this discipline. Incorporating the necessary components of pulmonary rehabilitation into the individual program will ensure comprehensive patient management. Setting goals for the patient and program will allow services to be individualized to meet the patient's unique needs. Finally, acceptance of a philosophy and code of ethics for pulmonary rehabilitation will ensure a patient-centered focus and continuous quality improvement.

Definition and Scope of Pulmonary Rehabilitation

Just as the conceptual background of pulmonary rehabilitation has changed over the years, its definition has evolved with time. A committee of the American College of Chest Physicians (ACCP) first defined pulmonary rehabilitation in 1974. In 1981 the American Thoracic Society (ATS) published the first official statement on pulmonary rehabilitation, which included the 1974 ACCP definition

of pulmonary rehabilitation.[9] In 1994 the National Institutes of Health (NIH) Consensus Conference on Pulmonary Rehabilitation formalized a definition of pulmonary rehabilitation.[10] The latest definition of pulmonary rehabilitation was published by the American Thoracic Society in 1999.[11] This definition, which is adopted by the Guidelines Committee of the AACVPR, is as follows:

> Pulmonary rehabilitation is a multidisciplinary program of care for patients with chronic respiratory impairment that is individually tailored and designed to optimize physical and social performance and autonomy.

Pulmonary rehabilitation is a component of standard medical care for patients with chronic respiratory diseases. Although it has little direct effect on the primary respiratory pathophysiological process, this form of therapy helps control and alleviate symptoms, optimizes functional capacity, improves health-related quality of life, and may reduce overall health care use. See figure 1.1 for the demonstrated outcomes of pulmonary rehabilitation. Although pulmonary rehabilitation has not been demonstrated to improve survival directly, studies to date have not had the statistical power to adequately test this. In all likelihood, pulmonary rehabilitation will favorably influence survival in some situations, such as in identifying significant

Figure 1.1 Demonstrated Outcomes of Pulmonary Rehabilitation

Reduced respiratory symptoms (e.g., dyspnea and fatigue)
Increased exercise performance
Increased knowledge about pulmonary disease and its management
Enhanced ability to perform activities of daily living
Improved health-related quality of life
Improved psychosocial symptoms (e.g., reversal of anxiety and depression, increased self-efficacy)
Reduced hospitalizations and use of medical resources
Return to work for some patients

Adapted, by permission, from A.L. Ries, 1990, "Position paper of the American Association of Cardiovascular and Pulmonary Rehabilitation: Scientific basis of pulmonary rehabilitation," *Journal of Cardiopulmonary Rehabilitation* 10: 418-441. © AACVPR.

hypoxemia and beginning long-term therapy with supplemental oxygen, and in educating patients to seek medical attention early in the course of an exacerbation of their respiratory disease.

Pulmonary rehabilitation works predominantly through reducing the effects of associated morbidity. An example of associated morbidity is the muscle wasting and weakness associated with COPD. Much of this associated morbidity is extremely treatable. Pulmonary rehabilitation services have been studied most extensively in patients with COPD but are also indicated for patients with other respiratory conditions, as detailed in chapter 7.

Complementing the strong scientific background, evidence, and rationale for pulmonary rehabilitation are the frequent patient testimonials. Subjective comments from patients provide further information and a sense of personal reality that enriches our knowledge and appreciation of the benefits of this therapy. An example of this is the following comment from a patient:

> Pulmonary rehabilitation has been a life-saving pathway between inactivity and activity, isolation and socialization, depression and hope, and from being an observer of life to an active participant.[12]

The Burden of Chronic Respiratory Disease

Since 1965 mortality from COPD in the United States has increased alarmingly. This increase in mortality is even more striking in light of the fact that the proportion of deaths from other common diseases, including coronary heart disease and stroke, are decreasing, as depicted in figure 1.2. Deaths from COPD are now ranked fourth, behind heart disease, stroke, and cancer (see figure 1.3). The death rate for women from COPD increased significantly compared with the increase in death rate for men. In 2000, for the first time in history, the number of women dying from COPD was greater than the number of men. "You've come a long way, baby" is not something we should be proud of as it relates to lung disease and death![13]

The National Health and Nutrition Examination Surveys III of 1991-1994 (NHANES III) estimated that 24 million adults in the United States had

Figure 1.3 Causes of Death in the United States	
Cause of death	**Number**
1. Heart disease	724,269
2. Cancer	538,947
3. Cerebrovascular disease (stroke)	158,060
4. Respiratory disease (COPD)	114,381
5. Accidents	94,828
6. Pneumonia and influenza	93,207
7. Diabetes	64,574
8. Suicide	29,264
9. Nephritis	26,295
10. Chronic liver disease	24,936
All other causes of death	469,314

From www.GOLDCOPD.com with permission.[14]

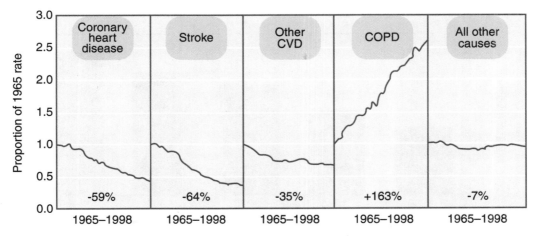

Figure 1.2   Percent change in age-adjusted death rates in the United States from 1965 to 1998.
From www.GOLDCOPD.com with permission.[14]

evidence of impaired lung function. In 2000 an estimated 10 million U.S. adults reported COPD, accounting for 8 million physician office visits for chronic and unspecified bronchitis, over 10 million physician office visits and hospital outpatient visits, 1.5 million emergency department visits, and 726,000 hospitalizations. Figure 1.4 depicts serial changes in health care use for airways disease from 1980 to 1998, reflecting this rise in the prevalence of chronic lung disease.

In 2001 the National Health Interview Survey estimated that 11.2 million Americans had chronic bronchitis, 3 million Americans had emphysema, and 14 to 15 million Americans had asthma. An estimated 6.3 million asthma sufferers were under the age of 18. The prevalence of, and mortality rate for, asthma has increased over all age groups. Between 1979 and 1998 the mortality rate for asthma increased 33% in males and 67% in females with the highest prevalence rate seen in children 5 to 17 years of age. Females had a higher rate than males. Females also have a death rate of 25% higher than men. Another alarming statistic is that death rates from asthma increased by 78% for children during that time.[15,16]

The economic cost of COPD in 1993 was $23.9 billion, including $14.7 billion for direct medical cost and an estimated $9.2 billion for indirect cost such as the loss of work time, a loss of productivity, and premature mortality. The economic cost of asthma was $12.7 billion—$8.1 billion for direct health care costs and $4.6 billion for indirect health care cost (lost productivity) with hospital services over $3.5 billion. The largest single indirect cost ($1.5 billion) was due to reduced productivity because of the loss of school days. Asthma is a serious chronic condition that accounts for about 3 million lost workdays for adults and 10.1 million lost school days for children

annually. In the past 20 years mortality, morbidity, and hospital discharge rates due to asthma have increased substantially. Asthma ranks within the top 10 prevalent conditions causing limitation of activity and cost to our nation.[13,16]

The impact of chronic respiratory disease is not just an economic or epidemiological statistic. Its effects on patients' and their families' quality of life is tremendous. The cost of lung disease in terms of lives affected is enormous.

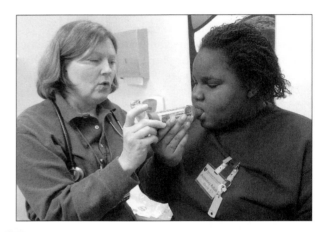

Asthma affects millions of people. Pulmonary rehabilitation can help lessen the effects of this and other respiratory illnesses.

A Brief History of Pulmonary Rehabilitation

The evolution of pulmonary rehabilitation to its current state follows the contributions of dedicated individuals and respected professional associations. To help us appreciate their contributions and the

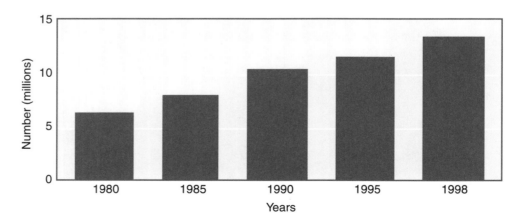

Figure 1.4 Changes in health care use for airways disease.

From www.GOLDCOPD.com with permission.[14]

resulting emergence of pulmonary rehabilitation as a respected scientific discipline, the following tables illustrate a few landmarks in the relatively brief history of pulmonary rehabilitation. Table 1.1 lists key scientific publications, and table 1.2 lists key events in the history of pulmonary rehabilitation.

Table 1.1 Key Publications in the History of Pulmonary Rehabilitation

Year	First author	Impact
1935	Livingston[17]	Presentation of the value of breathing exercises in asthma
1954	Miller[18]	Physiologic effects of diaphragmatic breathing in COPD
1956	Dayman[19]	Management of dyspnea in emphysema
1959	Barach[20]	Ambulatory oxygen therapy for chronic lung disease comes of age
1967	Miller[21]	Idea of rehabilitation for patients with COPD
1968	Celli[22]	Dyssynchronous breathing associated with arm but not leg exercise in patients with COPD
1969	Haas[23]	Rehabilitation in chronic obstructive pulmonary disease: a 5-year study of 252 male patients
1969	Petty[24]	Comprehensive care program for chronic airway obstruction, including many of the current principles of pulmonary rehabilitation
1970	Petty[25]	Ambulatory care for emphysema and chronic bronchitis, including more concepts of pulmonary rehabilitation
1971	Kass[26]	Nebraska COPD Rehabilitation Project: a multidisciplinary study identifying the factors involved in the rehabilitation of 140 patients with COPD
1973	Wasserman[27]	Classic book on exercise physiology in health and disease
1974	Hodgkin[28]	Further discussion on comprehensive care for COPD
1980	Nocturnal Oxygen Therapy Trial Group[29]	Established survival value of long-term supplemental oxygen use in hypoxemic patients with COPD
1980	Dudley[30]	Psychosocial concomitants to rehabilitation in COPD
1983	Bebout[31]	Clinical and physiological outcomes of a university hospital pulmonary rehabilitation program
1984	Mahler[32]	Introduction of the Baseline and Transition Dyspnea Indexes, which quantify dyspnea; have become valuable outcome measures
1987	Guyatt[33]	Introduction of the Chronic Respiratory Disease Questionnaire, now a widely used measure of health-related quality of life
1991	Casaburi[34]	First randomized trial showing the physiologic benefits of exercise training in COPD
1994	Reardon[35]	First randomized trial to show a beneficial effect of pulmonary rehabilitation on dyspnea
1994	Goldstein[36]	Randomized trial showing the benefits of pulmonary rehabilitation in multiple areas, including quality of life
1994	Ries[37]	Large randomized trial showing the positive effects of outpatient pulmonary rehabilitation on multiple outcomes over several years—a classic
1996	Lacasse[38]	A meta-analysis demonstrating the effectiveness of respiratory rehabilitation in COPD
1996	Maltais[39]	Study demonstrating that exercise training can improve skeletal muscle oxidative capacity in COPD patients
2000	Griffiths[40]	Large randomized trial of pulmonary rehabilitation that showed multiple benefits, including a reduction in health care use
2003	Bourbeau[41]	Study providing scientific evidence supporting the educational component of comprehensive pulmonary rehabilitation
2003	National Emphysema Treatment Trial (NETT) Research Group[42]	Pulmonary rehabilitation considered the "gold standard" of care: required before surgery and used as the therapy to which lung volume reduction surgery is compared

Table 1.2	Key Events in the History of Pulmonary Rehabilitation
Year	**Event**
1964	Smoking and Health: A Report of the Advisory Committee to the Surgeon General[43]
1974	A definition of pulmonary rehabilitation adopted by the American College of Chest Physicians and later quoted by the American Thoracic Society (1981)
1988	U.S. Surgeon General. The health consequences of smoking: Nicotine addiction[44]
1990	AACVPR position paper on the scientific basis of pulmonary rehabilitation[45]
1993	AACVPR's first published guidelines for pulmonary rehabilitation programs[46]
1994	National Institutes of Health workshop summary on pulmonary rehabilitation[47]
1995	ATS statement: Standards for the diagnosis and care of patients with chronic obstructive pulmonary disease[48]
1997	ACCP/AACVPR Pulmonary Rehabilitation Guidelines Panel: Evidence-based guidelines
1997	European Respiratory Society Task Force position paper: Selection criteria for pulmonary rehabilitation in COPD patients[49]
1998	AACVPR's second edition of guidelines for pulmonary rehabilitation programs
1998	National Lung Health Education Program (NLHEP)[50]
1997	Emphysema Treatment Trial Research Group, Rationale and design of the NETT trial[42]
1999	ATS official statement on pulmonary rehabilitation
1999	ATS. Dyspnea: Mechanisms, assessment and management: A consensus statement[51]
2000	AARC clinical practice guidelines for pulmonary rehabilitation[52]
2001	GOLD—Global Initiative for Chronic Obstructive Lung Disease
2001	British Thoracic Society Standards of Care Subcommittee on Pulmonary Rehabilitation[53]
2004	AACVPR's third edition of guidelines for pulmonary rehabilitation

Essential Components of Pulmonary Rehabilitation

The essential components of pulmonary rehabilitation are assessment, patient education and training, therapeutic exercise, psychosocial intervention, and the promotion of long-term adherence to its principles.[54,55,56] Prevention strategies and outcome assessment should be integrated into every aspect of the program. Outcome assessment will be reviewed in chapter 6.

As shown in figure 1.5, pulmonary rehabilitation is not simply an exercise or education program. Rather, it is an individualized program that meets the specific needs of the respiratory patient through all of the previously stated components. The pulmonary rehabilitation specialist must understand this concept when developing a complete and individualized therapeutic plan for the patient. The composition of the interdisciplinary team will

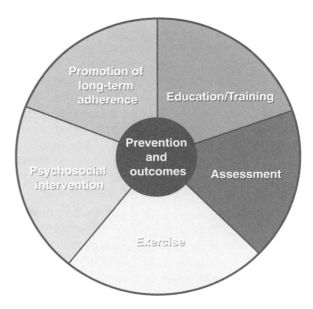

Figure 1.5 Essential components of pulmonary rehabilitation.

depend on the facility, resources, and patient needs (see chapter 8).

The significance of long-term adherence cannot be overstated. For patients to maintain and improve the benefits seen upon graduation from pulmonary rehabilitation, they must attend a maintenance exercise program, continue with the home recommendations or action plans they received upon discharge, or both. A significant portion of the educational component of pulmonary rehabilitation should be devoted to the promotion of long-term adherence. Patients experiencing an exacerbation of their respiratory disease are at special risk for becoming nonadherent with the ongoing maintenance plan. Long-term maintenance plans of pulmonary rehabilitation should provide mechanisms to facilitate a return to previously established rehabilitation plans following an exacerbation. This might involve having the patient return for short-term rehabilitation after exacerbation, when indicated. Ongoing communication among the patient, the physician, and the rehabilitation staff is essential.

Prevention

When people with chronic lung disease begin to seek medical attention, the underlying lung disease is often far advanced and has less potential for reversibility—although pulmonary rehabilitation can still provide substantial benefit in this situation. The onset of COPD is insidious, developing over 20 to 30 years with a long symptomatic period. During this period of time, early intervention, detection, and rehabilitation are critical. Even though the mean life expectancy in the United States, which was 77.2 years in 2001, continues to increase, people with advanced chronic lung disease will not have this favorable prognosis. Although people with advanced lung disease stand to improve with therapy such as pulmonary rehabilitation, logic dictates that they would experience greater improvement if their disease were identified and treated earlier. Understanding the natural course of chronic lung disease and the unique opportunity for intervention before a decline in lung function is paramount for the pulmonary rehabilitation specialist. Earlier detection and intervention would allow for preventive strategies such as smoking cessation, immunizations, adopting healthy lifestyles, and reducing environmental exposures. Getting a patient into pulmonary rehabilitation earlier in the course of the disease would also allow for greater levels of exercise training and would interrupt the vicious circle of inactivity, further deconditioning, and increasing dyspnea.[57,58]

The goal of earlier detection is not just for the COPD population but for any patient with chronic respiratory disease. Any person with a history of smoking, a family history of lung disease, a history of occupational or environmental exposures, and symptoms of cough and mucus production should automatically be considered for a spirometry test, which is considered the best assessment tool for

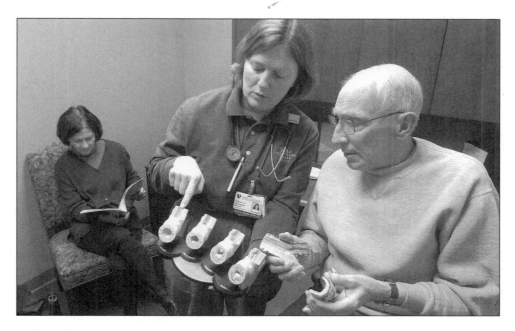

Smoking cessation classes are a must in any pulmonary rehabilitation program.

detecting lung abnormalities. To attack prevention, the motto "test your lungs, know your numbers" needs to be placed into action.[50]

The statistics that support the need for smoking cessation are overwhelming. In the United States in 1995, 24.7% of adults were smokers (47 million); of that number, 27% (24.5 million) were men and 22.6% (22.4 million) were women. An estimated 44.3 million adults are former smokers.[59] Every day in the United States 4,400 youths between the ages of 12 and 17 smoke their first cigarette. An estimated one third of these youths will die from a smoking-related disease. Between 2000 and 2003 the use of tobacco products in high school–age students decreased from 34.5% to 28.4%, but studies found no significant change among middle school–age students.[60] This is alarming. The prevention of tobacco use in our youth will reduce future smoking-related illnesses, including the costs and deaths associated with them.

Because quitting smoking has major and immediate health benefits for smokers of all ages, the inclusion of smoking cessation therapies (including the use of smokeless tobacco products) into every pulmonary rehabilitation service cannot be stressed enough. The excess risk of heart disease is reduced by half after 1 year of not smoking, after 10 years the risk of lung cancer drops to less than one half that of a continuing smoker, and in 5 to 15 years the risk of stroke returns to the level of those who never smoked. Even though irreversible lung disease may result from cigarette smoking, evidence suggests that the rate of decline of lung function in ex-smokers decreases to that of nonsmokers within a short period of time.

Pulmonary rehabilitation can complement the prevention strategies used by primary health care providers and specialists. The holistic approach of pulmonary rehabilitation is ideal for this facet of care.

Patient Goals

The patient and the pulmonary rehabilitation staff work jointly to develop short- and long-term goals during the course of the program. These are essential for the success of this therapy. Patient goals are established and reviewed with the patient and his or her significant other at the beginning of the program and then intermittently as needed. Goals should be realistic and achievable to improve patient motivation, adherence, and outcomes. It is important to note that individual patient goals may be altered as the program progresses and needs and expectations change. Following are some examples of patient goals:

- Breathe easier
- Be more active
- Have a better quality of life
- Increase strength and endurance
- Be able to perform activities of daily living, such as taking a shower or pursuing hobbies
- Be able to travel with greater ease
- Experience decreased anxiety, depression, or fear of activities that cause shortness of breath
- Experience fewer exacerbations and hospitalizations
- Be more independent and self-reliant
- Return to work
- Be able to clean house
- Be able to go to a movie

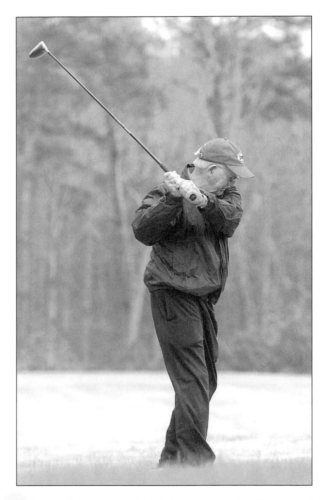

Being able to pursue hobbies is a great patient goal for rehabilitation programs.

The challenge of the pulmonary rehabilitation specialist is to translate these patient goals into a measurable format for assessment and documentation during the course of therapy.

Program Goals

Global program goals identify generalized approaches to holistic care. As such, they can be used to ensure the quality of the program and consistency across interdisciplinary team members. Following are examples of program goals:

- Integrate prevention and long-term adherence into the patient's treatment plan
- Design and implement an individualized therapeutic treatment plan (e.g., smoking cessation, weight loss or gain)
- Improve the patient's and his or her significant other's quality of life
- Control and alleviate, as much as possible, the symptoms and pathophysiological complications of respiratory impairment
- Increase strength, endurance, and exercise tolerance
- Decrease psychological symptoms such as anxiety or depression
- Increase the patient's long-term adherence with the medical and rehabilitation therapeutic treatment plan
- Train, motivate, and rehabilitate the patient to his or her maximum potential in self-care
- Train, motivate, and involve the patient's significant other in the patient's treatment plan
- Reduce the economic burden of pulmonary disease on society through a reduction of acute exacerbations, hospitalizations, lengths of stay, emergency room visits, and long-term convalescence
- Return the patient to gainful employment or active retirement if applicable
- Educate the general public and health care professionals about pulmonary health and rehabilitation
- Increase the medical community's awareness of the importance of early detection of pulmonary disease through screenings (e.g., spirometry)
- Increase the community's awareness of the harmful effects of smoking, nicotine addiction, and secondhand smoke, and of available treatment

Philosophy

Successful pulmonary rehabilitation requires that the patient, significant other, and interdisciplinary team members believe in the philosophy of pulmonary rehabilitation. This philosophy should include a belief in a rehabilitation therapeutic process that is centered on and developed in conjunction with the patient. As described in the code of ethics outlined in the following section, pulmonary rehabilitation team members should serve as role models in attitude, health, and professionalism.

Code of Ethics for the Pulmonary Rehabilitation Specialist

Pulmonary rehabilitation specialists involved in the care of patients with respiratory disease must strive, both individually and as a team, to maintain the highest ethical standards. The principles set forth in this document outline the ethical and moral standards to which each pulmonary rehabilitation specialist should conform.

The pulmonary rehabilitation specialist shall practice medically acceptable methods of pulmonary rehabilitation and shall not extend his or her practice beyond the competence and authority vested in him or her by state licensure, hospital policies and procedures, and the pulmonary rehabilitation medical director.

The pulmonary rehabilitation specialist shall always strive to increase and improve his or her knowledge expertise and render to each respiratory patient and significant other the full measure of his or her ability. All treatment modalities and services shall be provided with respect for the dignity of the patient and significant other, unrestricted by considerations of social, cultural, economic, personal, or religious beliefs.

The pulmonary rehabilitation specialist shall be responsible for the competent, efficient, and thorough performance of his or her designated duties.

The pulmonary rehabilitation specialist shall hold in strict confidence all patient information.

The pulmonary rehabilitation specialist, as a vital member of the interdisciplinary health care team, shall strive for the prevention and early detection, not just the treatment, of pulmonary disease.

Adapted, by permission, from the American Association for Respiratory Care, 1986, *Code of Ethics*. 11030 Ables Lane, Dallas, TX 75229.

Conclusion

Pulmonary rehabilitation is comprehensive and interdisciplinary, employs preventive and therapeutic treatment strategies, and is individualized to the patient's needs. Its importance is accentuated in light of the increasing prevalence of and morbidity attributed to chronic lung disease. Its primary goal is to restore or maintain an optimal level of physiological, psychological, social, occupational, and emotional function and well-being. It is well-documented that pulmonary rehabilitation leads to improvement in outcomes in multiple areas, including symptoms, exercise performance, functional status, and health status. Its essential components are assessment, patient education and training, therapeutic exercise, psychosocial intervention, and promotion of long-term adherence. Prevention and outcomes assessment should be integrated into all components. A formulation and understanding of the patient's goals will promote optimum care. Clearly stated program goals are necessary to ensure quality and consistency of care. Pulmonary rehabilitation is a standard of care for the symptomatic respiratory patient, complementing other standard medical therapies, such as pharmacologic therapy.

Selection and Assessment of the Pulmonary Rehabilitation Candidate

A comprehensive pulmonary rehabilitation program may be adapted for any person with chronic respiratory disease. The practice of reserving pulmonary rehabilitation for patients with end-stage respiratory disease or severe limitation of function results in many patients being denied the opportunity to benefit from this intervention. Therefore, pulmonary rehabilitation specialists need to educate the public and the medical community about the importance of the prevention and early detection of respiratory disease, as well as the rehabilitation of patients with respiratory disease.

The initial component of a pulmonary rehabilitation program is the interdisciplinary team assessment. This sets the foundation for all subsequent services provided during pulmonary rehabilitation, allowing for the development of the patient's individualized plan of care. This assessment is under the direction of the medical director and the program coordinator.

The components of patient education and training, exercise, and psychosocial interventions alone or together do not constitute pulmonary rehabilitation unless an initial and ongoing individualized assessment is included.

Patient Selection

A list of conditions considered appropriate for pulmonary rehabilitation is shown in figure 2.1. The degree of impairment noted in pulmonary function testing had been commonly used as the primary selection criterion in establishing patient eligibility for pulmonary rehabilitation. Although helpful in patient evaluation, pulmonary function test data are not sufficient as selection criteria alone. Symptoms, especially dyspnea, correlate better with functional ability than FEV_1 or other measures of pulmonary function.[1] In addition to the presence of disease, an important selection criterion should be a reduction in functional status or health-related quality of life resulting from the disease or its comorbidity. Symptoms, disability, and handicap despite standard medical therapy dictate the need for pulmonary rehabilitation, not the degree of physiologic impairment such as the FEV_1 or the diffusing capacity. Reductions in physical activity, occupational performance, and activities of daily living, and increases in medical resource consumption, should be evaluated and used in the selection process.[2,3]

In general, symptoms and functional status limitations from pulmonary disease become clinically apparent when one or more of the following objective tests reach the following levels of impairment:

- FEV_1 less than or equal to 65% of predicted
- FVC less than or equal to 65% of predicted
- Diffusing capacity for carbon monoxide adjusted for hemoglobin less than or equal to 65% of predicted
- Resting hypoxemia (S_aO_2/S_pO_2 less than or equal to 90%)
- Exercise testing demonstrating hypoxemia (S_aO_2/S_pO_2 less than or equal to 90%) or ventilatory limit ($\dot{V}E/MVV$ more than or equal to 0.8) or a rising Vd/Vt

However, for reasons described earlier, there are exceptions to these criteria, which are often related to prominent comorbidity. Conditions that commonly lead to referrals to pulmonary rehabilitation are listed in figure 2.2.

Figure 2.1 **Examples of Conditions Appropriate for Pulmonary Rehabilitation**

Obstructive Diseases
COPD (including alpha-1 antitrypsin deficiency)
Persistent asthma
Bronchiectasis
Cystic fibrosis
Bronchiolitis obliterans

Restrictive Diseases
Interstitial diseases
- Interstitial fibrosis
- Occupational or environmental lung disease
- Sarcoidosis
Chest wall diseases
- Kyphoscoliosis
- Ankylosing spondylitis
Neuromuscular diseases
- Parkinson's disease
- Postpolio syndrome
- Amyotrophic lateral sclerosis
- Diaphragmatic dysfunction
- Multiple sclerosis
- Posttuberculosis syndrome

Other Conditions
Lung cancer
Primary pulmonary hypertension
Pre and post thoracic and abdominal surgery
Pre and post lung transplantation
Pre and post lung volume reduction surgery
Ventilator dependency
Pediatric patients with respiratory disease
Obesity-related respiratory disease

Reprinted, by permission, from L. Beytas and G.L. Connors, 1993, Organization and management of a pulmonary rehabilitation program. In *Pulmonary rehabilitation: Guidelines to success*, 2nd ed., edited by J.E. Hodgkin, G.L. Connors, and C.W. Bell. Copyright 1993 by J.B. Lippincott.

Figure 2.2 **Conditions That Commonly Lead to Referrals to Pulmonary Rehabilitation**

Dyspnea/fatigue and chronic respiratory symptoms
Impaired health-related quality of life
Decreased functional status
Decreased occupational performance
Difficulty performing activities of daily living
Difficulty with the medical regimen
Psychosocial problems attendant to the underlying respiratory illness
Nutritional depletion
Increased use of medical resources (e.g., hospitalizations, emergency room visits, physician visits)
Gas exchange abnormalities including hypoxemia

Concurrent diseases or conditions that may interfere with the rehabilitation process or place the patient at substantial risk during exercise should be corrected or stabilized before the patient enters the program. Permanent or temporary conditions that may be considered contraindications to pulmonary rehabilitation include, but are not limited to, unstable cardiac disease and severe pulmonary hypertension. Stable cardiac disease, with a practitioner's clearance, is not a contraindication to pulmonary rehabilitation. Other disease states that may require modification of the program include advanced liver disease, stroke, cognitive deficit, and psychiatric disease. The clinical judgments of the medical director and rehabilitation team during the initial assessment are necessary for determining whether this comorbidity would preclude pulmonary rehabilitation.

The concomitant use of tobacco in patients beginning pulmonary rehabilitation is a controversial issue. Some programs exclude actively smoking patients from participating in pulmonary rehabilitation, believing they are less motivated and committed than the nonsmoker or ex-smoker. This belief has not been substantiated, and cigarette smokers may in fact be more in need of rehabilitation than nonsmokers. If active smokers are accepted, smoking cessation is a major component and goal of the rehabilitation process.

Patient motivation is also a necessary consideration in patient selection, although it is difficult to assess. Patients must agree to commit to complete the program and be active participants. Patients who initially appear resistant to rehabilitation, however, often show dramatic improvement and become advocates of the program. Therefore, patient motivation should not be considered too strongly in the evaluation criteria.

Discussing the patient's financial ability to meet the anticipated expenses of pulmonary rehabilitation is necessary. Third-party payers should be contacted to determine if the rehabilitation program is a covered benefit and if so, to what extent. Patients are then able to determine if they can afford the out-of-pocket expenses. Verbal and written information regarding program fees and coverage must be given to the patient prior to admission.

Patients being considered must also have a means of transportation to and from the program. This may be provided by family members, friends, or public transit. Local and regional telephone books have transportation assistance information available from state and federal agencies. It is often listed under "disabled," "handicapped," or "aging" headings.

Patients too ill to attend outpatient pulmonary rehabilitation regularly may be more appropriate candidates for admission to an inpatient rehabilitation facility or home care. If the pulmonary rehabilitation facility has a social services department, the staff of that department may assist patients with financial issues, transportation, and access to community support networks.

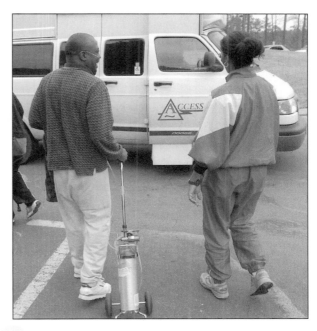

Patients must be able to get to pulmonary rehabilitation classes. Public transportation is one way for older patients to get to program sites.

Patient Assessment

The initial pulmonary rehabilitation assessment and reassessment is performed by the program coordinator or trained health care designee and appropriate team members. This assessment sets the foundation for all services of the interdisciplinary team provided during pulmonary rehabilitation, allowing the development of the patient's individualized plan of care. The initial assessment should include a patient interview and the components listed in figure 2.3. These assessments may be performed by various members of the interdisciplinary team, as determined by the patient's individualized needs. An in-depth interview with the patient and family or significant other is necessary in order to help assess the patient and to establish appropriate individual goals.[4,5] A sample initial interview form can be found in appendix A. Another approach to

Figure 2.3   Components of the Initial Patient Assessment

Patient interview
Medical history and physical exam
Diagnostic tests
Symptoms assessment
Musculoskeletal and exercise assessment
Activities of daily living assessment
Nutritional assessment
Educational assessment
Psychosocial assessment
Goal development

obtaining patient information is to request that the patient complete a questionnaire prior to the interview. A sample questionnaire can be found in appendix A.

The importance of the initial interview cannot be overstated. Not only are assessments made and goals formulated, but also the foundations of trust and credibility are generated at this time. The interview allows the patient to interact on a personal level with the rehabilitation staff, see where the program is located, and possibly meet rehabilitation graduates.

Medical History

A thorough review of the patient's medical status is essential for the initial assessment. Much of this information can be obtained from patient records in the physician's office or the hospital. The medical history is important in highlighting comorbid conditions that may have a direct bearing on the patient's health, well-being, and progress in the pulmonary rehabilitation program. One example is a patient with a hip or knee disorder who may need to have the frequency, intensity, and mode of exercise adjusted. It is often useful for the pulmonary rehabilitation staff to communicate with the referring physician to determine the principal factors that are contributing to the patient's symptoms and functional limitation. A sample physician referral form can be found in appendix A. Following is a list of the medical history information to be gathered:

Components of the Medical History

- Respiratory history
- Active medical problems or comorbidities
- Other medical and surgical history
- Family history of respiratory disease
- Use of medical resources (e.g., hospitalizations, urgent care or emergency room visits, physician visits)
- All current medications including over-the-counter drugs and herbal supplements
- Allergies and drug intolerance
- Smoking history
- Occupational, environmental, and recreational exposures
- Alcohol and other substance abuse history

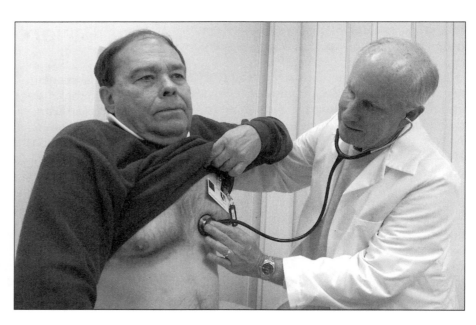

It's important to make sure a patient has a thorough physical assessment before the start of a rehabilitation program. This assessment can identify any problem areas the patient may have.

Physical Assessment

Physical assessment includes examining the chest and measuring and evaluating vital signs, the use of accessory muscles of respiration, finger clubbing, edema, and other signs of heart failure such as jugular venous distention.[6] Measurement of arterial oxygen saturation with pulse oximetry at rest and with activity is frequently performed during the initial physical assessment. The physical assessment represents a simple and noninvasive way to evaluate, monitor, and follow the patient's progress. Following is a list of the components of the physical assessment:

Focused Physical Assessment

- Vital signs: height, weight, blood pressure, heart rate, respiratory rate, temperature
- Breathing pattern
- Use of accessory muscles of respiration
- Chest examination: inspection, palpation, percussion, symmetry, diaphragm position, breath sounds, duration of expiratory phase, forced expiratory time, adventitial sounds
- Signs of heart disease: S3 gallop, bibasilar lung crackles, peripheral edema, jugular venous distention, heart murmurs
- Presence of finger clubbing
- Arterial oxygen saturation measured with pulse oximetry at rest and with activity
- Upper and lower extremity evaluation: signs of vascular insufficiency, joint disease, musculoskeletal dysfunction

Diagnostic Tests

Essential diagnostic information to assist in the proper diagnosis of the rehabilitation candidate and the development of an appropriate plan of care is listed in figure 2.4.[7] These diagnostic tests identify the patient's disease(s) and establish a baseline of the patient's current clinical status and may be used postprogram to evaluate outcomes. The additional laboratory tests listed in figure 2.5 may also be helpful for selected patients as determined by the initial and ongoing assessments.

Symptom Assessment

Dyspnea and fatigue are primary symptoms in patients with respiratory disease and must be documented and quantified. Onset, quality, quantity, frequency, and duration are often used to describe symptoms. In addition, identifying and alleviating

---

Figure 2.4 Essential Diagnostic Data Needed for the Initial Medical Evaluation of the Pulmonary Rehabilitation Candidate

Spirometry
Oxygen saturation at rest and with walking exercise upon program entry
Chest radiograph
Electrocardiogram
Field test of exercise capacity, such as the 6-minute walk test or the shuttle walk test, upon program entry
Screening assessment of anxiety and depression, such as the Beck Depression Inventory or the Hospital Anxiety and Depression Questionnaire, upon program entry
CBC

Figure 2.5 Diagnostic Medical Tests to Consider for Selected Patients

Complete pulmonary function test (spirometry, lung volumes, diffusing capacity)
Maximal inspiratory and expiratory pressures
Cardiopulmonary exercise testing
Complex metabolic study (measurement of expired gases)
Simple symptom-limited exercise study
Bone density measurement
Gastroesophageal reflux testing
Dysphagia evaluation
Bronchial challenge
Postexercise spirometry
Cardiovascular testing: Holter monitor, echocardiogram, thallium exercise stress test
Sleep study
Sinus radiographs
Complete blood count and blood chemistry
Theophylline level
Alpha-1 antitrypsin determination
Skin tests

---

irritating factors is important. Information from symptom assessment may be used to document outcomes and is often used by third-party payers to determine the medical necessity for payment authorization. Following is a list of items to include in the symptom assessment:

Symptom Assessment

- Dyspnea: on exertion, paroxysmal, at rest, nocturnal
- Fatigue
- Cough
- Sputum volume, color, consistency, smell
- Wheeze
- Hemoptysis
- Chest pain
- Postnasal drainage
- Reflux, heartburn
- Edema: pedal, pretibial
- Dysphagia, swallowing problems
- Extremity pain or weakness

An objective rating of dyspnea is crucial in the assessment because it is usually the overriding symptom in respiratory disease and is reduced by pulmonary rehabilitation.[1] Dyspnea during exercise is commonly rated with a 10-point Borg scale or a visual analog scale. These two methods of rating dyspnea are explained in chapter 4. The impact of dyspnea on physical function can be measured with the Baseline Dyspnea Index (BDI), the Medical Research Council Scale (MRC), the Oxygen Cost Diagram (OCD), the UCSD shortness of breath questionnaire (SOBQ), or the dyspnea domain of the Chronic Respiratory Disease Questionnaire (CRQ, or CRDQ). These are discussed in chapter 6.

Musculoskeletal and Exercise Assessment

The safety of an exercise training program and the appropriateness of the exercise prescription are determined by a thorough initial musculoskeletal and exercise assessment. This assessment includes evaluation of the patient's exercise tolerance, physical limitations, and requirements for supplemental oxygen. An evaluation of gait and balance should also be included in the assessment. A sample physical therapy evaluation form can be found in appendix A.

The assessment of physical limitations serves to establish a baseline of strength, range of motion, posture, functional abilities, and activities.[8,9] The evaluation should also address orthopedic limitations, any activity restrictions requiring exercise modification, and transferring abilities such as from a chair to a standing position or from the floor to a standing position. See chapter 4 for a detailed description of an exercise assessment. Following is a list of the information to be obtained in the exercise assessment:

Exercise Assessment

- Physical limitations (e.g., strength, range of motion, posture, functional abilities, and activities)
- Orthopedic limitations
- Transferring abilities
- Exercise tolerance: timed distance walk test or shuttle walk test
- Exercise hypoxemia including the need for supplemental oxygen therapy
- Gait and balance
- Exercise modification

Pain Assessment

Assessing pain during the initial assessment and during daily sessions throughout the exercise program is also necessary. Parameters to be assessed include location, duration, intensity, and character. Intensity is usually rated on a 0 to 10 scale or a facial descriptor scale. Assessment also must include factors that aggravate or ameliorate the pain.

Activities of Daily Living Assessment

Dyspnea often leads to a decreased ability and willingness to perform activities of daily living (ADLs); therefore, the patient's ability to function independently in ADLs and leisure activities should be assessed. The ADL assessment should include energy conservation techniques, extremity strength and range of motion, proper breathing techniques with daily activities, and the need for adaptive equipment.[10] If appropriate, functional task performance and the work environment's demands should be assessed to establish a baseline for planning treatment and measuring outcomes. Appendix A lists levels of energy expenditure for common household and leisure activities (in METs) that may be used as a tool to assess patients' ability to perform ADLs. An interview with a significant other frequently adds complementary information to the patient's self-report.

Sexual dysfunction resulting from chronic pulmonary disease is another important area to be assessed.[11] See chapter 5 for additional information on sexuality. Understanding the patient's concerns and previous patterns of sexual activity will help in

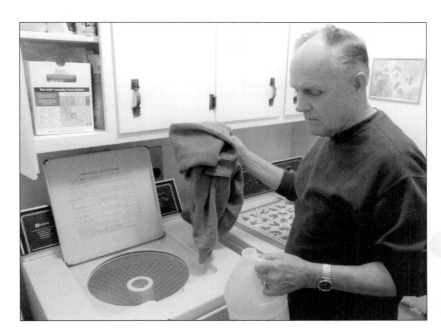

Activities of daily living include such tasks as doing laundry and fixing meals. It's important to assess a patient's level of activity of daily living before starting a rehabilitation program.

the plan for counseling, if necessary. The reaction of the significant other to the disease and its effect on mutual sexual function is important to determine. Following is a list of the information to be obtained in the ADL assessment:

ADL Assessment

- Functional task performance, which may include a formal functional capacity assessment
- Breathing techniques with ADLs
- Extremity function
- Energy conservation
- Need for adaptive equipment
- Food procurement and preparation
- Leisure impairment
- Sexual function
- Vocational evaluation

Nutritional Assessment

Patients with respiratory disease often have significant alterations in nutritional status and body composition.[12] Chronic respiratory disease causes increased energy expenditure during breathing, which results in increased caloric needs.[13] Problems maintaining adequate nutrition are present in 40% to 60% of patients with COPD,[14] and poor nutritional status is a significant, independent predictor of mortality.[15] Weight gain is indicated for the underweight patient. Patients who are overweight possibly as a result of inactivity or medications require a weight loss program. These patients experience an increase in their work of breathing and shortness of breath as a result of being overweight.

Minimal nutritional assessment includes measurement of height and weight, calculation of body mass index (BMI, see table 2.1), and documentation of recent weight change. In addition, fluid intake and alcohol consumption should be recorded. A sample nutritional assessment can be found in appendix A. Other assessments should be based on the needs of the patient. Following is a list of items included in the nutritional assessment:

Nutritional Assessment

- Height and weight
- Body mass index (BMI)
- Weight change
- Dietary history, eating patterns, diet recall (3 days), dietary journal when appropriate
- Person responsible for shopping and food preparation
- Fluid intake
- Alcohol consumption
- Laboratory tests of nutritional status: serum albumin, prealbumin
- Drug–nutrient interactions
- Lean body mass determination, when indicated
- Need for nutritional supplements

Table 2.1 Body Mass Index

BMI	19	20	21	22	23	24	25	26	27	28	29	30	31	32	33	34	35
Height (inches)	Body Weight (pounds)																
	Normal						Overweight					Obese					
58	91	96	100	105	110	115	119	124	129	134	138	143	148	153	158	162	167
59	94	99	104	109	114	119	124	128	133	138	143	148	153	158	163	168	173
60	97	102	107	112	118	123	128	133	138	143	148	153	158	163	168	174	179
61	100	106	111	116	122	127	132	137	143	148	153	158	164	169	174	180	185
62	104	109	115	120	126	131	136	142	147	153	158	164	169	175	180	186	191
63	107	113	118	124	130	135	141	146	152	158	163	169	175	180	186	191	197
64	110	116	122	128	134	140	145	151	157	163	169	174	180	186	192	197	204
65	114	120	126	132	138	144	150	156	162	168	174	180	186	192	198	204	210
66	118	124	130	136	142	148	155	161	167	173	179	186	192	198	204	210	216
67	121	127	134	140	146	153	159	166	172	178	185	191	198	204	211	217	223
68	125	131	138	144	151	158	164	171	177	184	190	197	203	210	216	223	230
69	128	135	142	149	155	162	169	176	182	189	196	203	209	216	223	230	236
70	132	139	146	153	160	167	174	181	188	195	202	209	216	222	229	236	243
71	136	143	150	157	165	172	179	186	193	200	208	215	222	229	236	243	250
72	140	147	154	162	169	177	184	191	199	206	213	221	228	235	242	250	258
73	144	151	159	166	174	182	189	197	204	212	219	227	235	242	250	257	265
74	148	155	163	171	179	186	194	202	210	218	225	233	241	249	256	264	272
75	152	160	168	176	184	192	200	208	216	224	232	240	248	256	264	272	279
76	156	164	172	180	189	197	205	213	221	230	238	246	254	263	271	279	287

Adapted from *Clinical Guidelines on the Identification, Evaluation, and Treatment of Overweight and Obesity in Adults: The Evidence Report.* www.nhlbi.nih.gov/guidelines/obesity/bmi_tbl.htm

- Use of nutritional or herbal supplements
- Dentition and mastication

Educational Assessment

Patients' knowledge of the level of their individual disease process and the strategies they use to cope with their illness can be measured during the initial assessment. This can provide a baseline for evaluating change in knowledge as a result of the program, and is a method of documenting outcomes. An example of a pretest used for assessing the patient's knowledge and an education log are shown in appendix A. A number of areas in addition to patients' knowledge of their disease should be evaluated,[16] including the ability to read or write, hearing or vision impairment, cognitive impairment, language barriers, and cultural diversity (ethnicity, cultural beliefs, and customs). This information can be ascertained during the initial interview session. See chapter 3 for further information on how to develop an educational plan. Following is a list of items included in the educational assessment:

Educational Assessment

- Knowledge of disease and its treatment
- Hearing
- Vision
- Cognitive ability

36	37	38	39	40	41	42	43	44	45	46	47	48	49	50	51	52	53	54
Body Weight (pounds)																		
Obese				Extreme Obesity														
172	177	181	186	191	196	201	205	210	215	220	224	229	234	239	244	248	253	258
178	183	188	193	198	203	208	212	217	222	227	232	237	242	247	252	257	262	267
184	189	194	199	204	209	215	220	225	230	235	240	245	250	255	261	266	271	276
190	195	201	206	211	217	222	227	232	238	243	248	254	259	264	269	275	280	285
196	202	207	213	218	224	229	235	240	246	251	256	262	267	273	278	284	289	295
203	208	214	220	225	231	237	242	248	254	259	265	270	278	282	287	293	299	304
209	215	221	227	232	238	244	250	256	262	267	273	279	285	291	296	302	308	314
216	222	228	234	240	246	252	258	264	270	276	282	288	294	300	306	312	318	324
223	229	235	241	247	253	260	266	272	278	284	291	297	303	309	315	322	328	334
230	236	242	249	255	261	268	274	280	287	293	299	306	312	319	325	331	338	344
236	243	249	256	262	269	276	282	289	295	302	308	315	322	328	335	341	348	354
243	250	257	263	270	277	284	291	297	304	311	318	324	331	338	345	351	358	365
250	257	264	271	278	285	292	299	306	313	320	327	334	341	348	355	362	369	376
257	265	272	279	286	293	301	308	315	322	329	338	343	351	358	365	372	379	386
265	272	279	287	294	302	309	316	324	331	338	346	353	361	368	375	383	390	397
272	280	288	295	302	310	318	325	333	340	348	355	363	371	378	386	393	401	408
280	287	295	303	311	319	326	334	342	350	358	365	373	381	389	396	404	412	420
287	295	303	311	319	327	335	343	351	359	367	375	383	391	399	407	415	423	431
295	304	312	320	328	336	344	353	361	369	377	385	394	402	410	418	426	435	443

- Language
- Literacy
- Cultural diversity

Psychosocial Assessment

Routine psychosocial assessment is an integral component of pulmonary rehabilitation. This initially involves clinical assessment by the pulmonary rehabilitation team, aided by the use of screening questionnaires that assess anxiety and depression. Patients identified with significant psychosocial problems are referred for further evaluation (and, if indicated, treatment) to appropriate professionals, such as a clinical social worker, psychiatric nurse, psychologist, or psychiatrist. The psychosocial assessment should address several areas: motivation level, emotional distress, substance abuse, cognitive impairment, interpersonal conflict, other psychopathology (e.g., depression, anxiety), significant neuropsychological impairment (e.g., memory, attention and concentration, problem-solving impairments during daily activities), coping style, and sexual dysfunction. Failure to detect the presence of significant psychosocial pathology may result in poor progress with rehabilitation. The findings from the psychosocial assessment are most useful if they lead to specific and individually tailored treatment goals and are integrated into the overall interdisciplinary treatment plan.

In general, psychosocial evaluation and treatment should be integrated into every component of pulmonary rehabilitation from assessment through follow-up. Psychosocial assessment is covered in detail in chapter 5. Following is a list of items included in the psychosocial assessment:

Psychosocial Assessment

- Perception of quality of life and ability to adjust to the disease
- Interpersonal conflict
- Anxiety and depression
- Substance abuse
- Addictive disorders
- Neuropsychological impairment
- Sexual dysfunction
- Motivation for pulmonary rehabilitation

Goal Development

Goal development is a direct reflection of the potential of the rehabilitation candidate. Goal development must include short-term and long-term individual patient goals. Program goals must incorporate and reflect these individual patient goals. Measurable, patient-specific goals are formulated from data collected during the initial patient assessment. Setting realistic goals that are compatible with the patient's underlying disease, the patient's needs and expectations, and the program's objectives is important. Goals should be formulated with the patient. Examples include the ability to return to work, care for family, walk to the mailbox, bowl, play golf, perform proper breathing techniques, and better understand the disease and its therapy. The patient must have a clear understanding of the goals and should agree to work toward their attainment. Reviewing progress toward goals throughout the program facilitates their attainment. Involving significant others in the goal-setting process at the beginning of the program helps to ensure that everyone understands what can and cannot be expected as a result of the program.

Rehabilitation Potential

At the completion of the comprehensive assessment, the patient's rehabilitation potential must be ascertained. Categorization into poor, fair, good, and excellent potential can then be made based on the assessment information. This categorization is at best arbitrary because mitigating factors such as poor motivation can improve with the rehabilitation process. The clinical judgment of the pulmonary rehabilitation team aids in this determination.

Conclusion

In the patient selection process, pulmonary rehabilitation is indicated for any patient who remains symptomatic or who is impaired in the ability to perform ADLs as a result of chronic respiratory disease. Assessment of the pulmonary rehabilitation patient by an interdisciplinary team sets the foundation for an individualized and comprehensive pulmonary rehabilitation program. Assessment is one of the most critical components of a program; it is a precursor to patient education and training, psychosocial intervention, exercise, and follow-up. Realistic patient goals are determined during the assessment and reevaluated during the program as necessary.

Assessment is the cornerstone to optimal outcomes and the effectiveness of pulmonary rehabilitation and may also prevent potential complications of chronic respiratory disease.

Patient Education and Skills Training

The objective of patient education and skills training is to encourage behavioral change that leads to improved health and a commitment to long-term adherence. Patients who fully participate in this aspect of pulmonary rehabilitation become more active participants in their own health care.[1,2] Upon completion of a thorough assessment, the interdisciplinary team can then begin to develop the necessary education and training sessions. Achieving the goals of pulmonary rehabilitation requires that the patient and a support person understand the underlying pulmonary disorder and the principles of self-management. This requires guidance from the interdisciplinary team.[3,4] The process of behavioral change is ongoing and is achieved through providing a strong foundation that allows patients to build on their knowledge. This chapter discusses the basic principles of patient education and skills training that should be included in the curriculum of pulmonary rehabilitation.

Education Process

Key steps in the education process include the following:

- Assessing the patient's educational needs (see chapter 2)
- Determining how the patient learns best
- Selecting the approach or style that most benefits the patient

When developing an individualized teaching plan, the patient's age, cultural background, language, educational level, and previous life experiences must be incorporated.[5,6] No single approach or style of learning is best, but repetition, straightforwardness, and mutual respect are key aspects in achieving successful learning. Pulmonary rehabilitation educators should present the material in an organized sequence using appropriate terminology, document the education and training sessions, and determine the reinforcement and follow-up needed.

The majority of patients who enter pulmonary rehabilitation have not been in a formal classroom situation for many years. Educators need to create a comfortable and relaxed environment that will allow these patients to become at ease with the setting and the material taught. Everyone learns differently, but a patient's retention of material can be improved by the way the information is presented.

Patients acquire new information through visual, auditory, and tactile senses, and through the use of psychomotor skills (hands-on learning).[7] Figure 3.1 illustrates the importance of including the acts of hearing, seeing, and doing in curriculum development. In an educational and skills training program, team members should use each of these processes

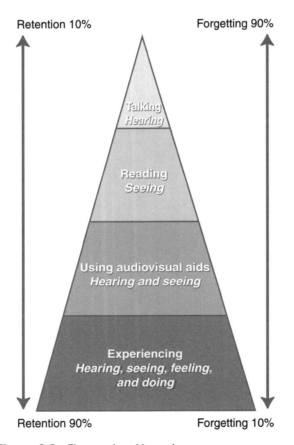

Figure 3.1 The scale of learning.

Reprinted, by permission, from J.W. Hopp and S.E. Maddox, 1984, Education of patients and their families. In *Pulmonary rehabilitation: Guidelines to success*, edited by J.E. Hodgkin, E.G. Zorn, and G.L. Connors. Copyright 1984 by J.E. Hodgkin.

to improve patients' ability to retain newly learned material. Interdisciplinary team members can improve their communication style by making sure they face the patient, get the patient's attention, leave their faces or mouths uncovered when talking, do not face away from the patient when speaking (especially when writing on a board or flipchart), speak in a volume that is neither too loud nor too soft, speak slowly, and articulate as clearly as possible. Background noise, inadequate lighting, distractions, sound reverberation, poor seating arrangement, and too great a distance between the speaker and listener should be avoided.

Providing written material such as an education manual improves comprehension and retention of the considerable amount of information presented during pulmonary rehabilitation. This manual is an important resource for the patient and significant other(s) throughout the program and following graduation (see figure 3.2 for a sample table of contents). When developing or selecting the written materials for the education and skills training sessions, consider the following: the reading level of the patient,[8] visual or hearing impairments, language barriers, cultural differences,[9] and cognitive impairments.

Focus and Scope of Educational and Skills Training

A primary objective of pulmonary rehabilitation education and training is to achieve optimal levels of understanding and self-management. This will be reflected in achieving maximal function, transfer of gains to the home setting, long-term adherence, and a reduction in dependency.[10] Educational needs are determined during the initial evaluation and should be reassessed during the program. Interdisciplinary team members with special training or expertise in a particular content area should present the relevant information at the education and skills training sessions. Many excellent education and training resources are available for content development (e.g., AACVPR educational resources, medical textbooks).[11-17] Figure 3.3 lists a sample of Internet sites that provide staff and patient educational information.

Depending on the patient's individual needs, any or all of the following topics may be included in the education and skills training component of pulmonary rehabilitation:

1) Normal Pulmonary Anatomy and Physiology

2) Chronic Lung Disease
   a) COPD
   b) Chronic Bronchitis
   c) Emphysema
   d) Asthma
   e) Bronchiectasis
   f) Restrictive Lung Disease
   g) Other Conditions

3) Description and Interpretation of Medical Tests
   a) Spirometry
   b) Lung Volumes
   c) Pulse Oximetry
   d) Arterial Blood Gas
   e) Other

4) Breathing Retraining
   a) Pursed-Lip Breathing
   b) Abdominal Breathing
   c) Application of Breathing Strategies to Panic Control

5) Bronchial Hygiene
   a) Cough Techniques
   b) Postural Drainage
   c) Positive Airway Pressure

6) Medications
   a) Oxygen
   b) Proper Inhaler Technique
      i) Metered-Dose Inhaler
      ii) Dry Powder Inhaler
      iii) Use of Spacer Chamber
   c) Bronchodilators
      i) Oral
      ii) Inhaled
   d) Steroids
      i) Oral
      ii) Inhaled
   e) Antibiotics
   f) Tranquilizers and Sedatives
   g) Diuretics

7) Benefits of Exercise
   a) General Principles
      i) Aerobic
      ii) Strength
   b) Home Exercise Program

8) Activities of Daily Living (ADLs)
   a) Breathing Strategies During ADLs
   b) Energy Conservation
   c) Work Simplification

9) Eating Right
   a) General Nutrition Guidelines
   b) Strategies for Weight Loss
   c) Strategies for Weight Gain

10) Irritant Avoidance/Prevention and Control of Respiratory Infections
    a) Smoking Cessation
       i) Importance and Benefits
       ii) Techniques
       iii) Resources
    b) Hazards of Secondhand Smoke
    c) Environmental and Occupational Irritant Avoidance
    d) Signs and Symptoms of a Respiratory Infection
    e) When to Call Your Health Care Provider
    f) Self-Management Strategies for Increased Symptoms
    g) Vaccinations

11) Leisure Activities
    a) Travel
       i) Availability of Oxygen
    b) Sexuality

12) Coping With Chronic Lung Disease and End-of-Life Planning
    a) Depression Management
    b) Panic Control
    c) Patient–Caregiver Relationship
    d) Advance Directive Planning
       i) Importance of Patient–Physician–Family Discussion
       ii) Durable Power of Attorney for Health Care
       iii) Living Will
       iv) Prehospital Medical Care Directive

Figure 3.2 Sample table of contents from a patient manual.

Web Site Address	Sponsor
www.airwavesonline.com	Boehringer Ingelheim Pharmaceuticals, Inc.
www.thebreathingspace.com	Boehringer Ingelheim Pharmaceuticals, Inc.
www.mayoclinic.com	Mayo Foundation for Medical Education and Research
www.healthfinder.gov	Office of Disease Prevention and Health Promotion, U.S. Department of Health and Human Services
www.vh.org	Virtual Hospital, University of Iowa
www.lungusa.org	American Lung Association
www.nhlbi.nih.gov	National Heart, Lung, and Blood Institute, National Institutes of Health
www.alpha1.org	Alpha-1 Association
www.lung.ca	Canadian Lung Association
www.oxygen4travel.com	Guide for Travelers with Pulmonary Disabilities
www.nationaljewish.org	National Jewish Medical and Research Center
www.nlhep.org	National Lung Health Education Program
www.aarc.org	American Association for Respiratory Care
www.chestnet.org	American College of Chest Physicians
www.thoracic.org	American Thoracic Society
www.noah-health.org	New York Online Access to Health
www.cff.org	Cystic Fibrosis Foundation
www.cdc.gov	Centers for Disease Control and Prevention, U.S. Department of Health and Human Services

Figure 3.3 Internet sites that provide staff and patient educational materials.

- Normal pulmonary anatomy and physiology
- Pathophysiology of lung disease
- Description and interpretation of medical tests
- Breathing retraining
- Bronchial hygiene
- Medications including oxygen
- Exercise principles
- Activities of daily living (ADLs) and energy conservation
- Respiratory modalities
- Self-assessment and symptom management
- Nutrition
- Psychosocial issues
- Ethical issues
- Advance directives

Refer to figure 3.4 for a sample form that may be used for the documentation of educational interventions and outcomes.

Normal Pulmonary Anatomy and Physiology

Presenting the anatomy and physiology of the respiratory system in a simple and basic way is important in pulmonary rehabilitation. It sets the groundwork for understanding respiratory illness. It is particularly useful to use demonstration models and other teaching aids when discussing this material because laypersons frequently have difficulty envisioning the pulmonary anatomy.

Pathophysiology of Lung Disease

Content discussed regarding the pathophysiology of the patient's disease should be tailored to mirror the diagnosis that the patient has received from his or her physician. With a basic understanding of their specific respiratory disease, most patients are more willing to comply with their prescribed therapeutic interventions.

Patient name: _____

Medical record #: _____

Diaphragmatic and Pursed-Lip Breathing (DB/PLB)

	Goals	Objectives	Assessment	Outcome
Session I	Instruct on anatomy and physiology of normal lung disease process, and the effect of bronchial collapse.	Identify the effects of bronchial collapse; increase O_2 saturation during technique.	Written or verbal review. Participant identified effects of bronchial collapse and O_2 saturation pre- and post-PLB.	Met Not met Date __ ____ ___ Comments: _____ _____ _____ Sig:_____
Session II	Instruct and demonstrate the proper techniques of DB/PLB.	Will be able to demonstrate the proper techniques of DB/PLB while usng a _____-lb weight on abdomen while lying, if there are no contraindications.	Participant demonstrated proper DB/PLB technique with _____-lb weight on abdomen.	Met Not met Date __ ____ ___ Comments: _____ _____ _____ Sig:_____
Session III	Instruct and demonstrate the use of DB/PLB with activities of daily living.	Will be able to demonstrate the proper use of DB/PLB while performing activities of daily living.	Participant demonstrated proper DB/PLB technique with activities of daily living.	Met Not met Date __ ____ ___ Comments: _____ _____ _____ Sig:_____
Session IV	Instruct on the benefits of using DB/PLB for panic control.	Will be able to verbally explain and identify the importance and purpose of DB/PLB for panic control.	Given written or verbal review questions. Participant gave correct response on the purpose of using DB/PLB for panic control.	Met Not met Date __ ____ ___ Comments: _____ _____ _____ Sig:_____

Figure 3.4   Example of pulmonary rehabilitation progress notes for diaphragmatic and pursed-lip breathing.

Adapted from Missouri Baptist Medical Center Pulmonary Rehabilitation Program, St. Louis, Missouri.

Medical Tests

Because the description and interpretation of medical tests can be very confusing to the patient, explanations should be kept simple. Many times patients have never seen their test results, nor have they understood how their results compare to the normal range. The patient's ability to understand the medical tests and the results can facilitate adherence with the treatment plans. This education should supplement the information given in the medical office. Following are some of the medical tests that might be discussed with patients:

- Timed distance walk test[18]
- Pulmonary function tests[19]
- Cardiopulmonary stress test [20]
- Arterial blood gases[21]
- Pulse oximetry [22, 23]
- Chest X ray
- Electrocardiogram
- Complete blood count/electrolytes
- Sleep study

Breathing Retraining

It is important to teach every patient proper breathing techniques. Diaphragmatic and pursed-lip breathing may help patients control and relieve

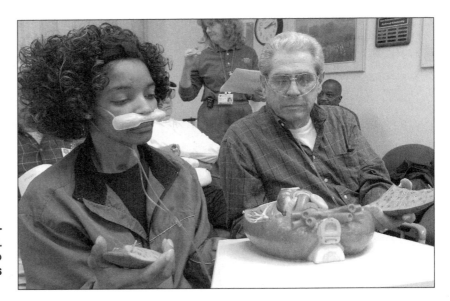

Models are an important teaching tool in rehabilitation programs. Models allow patients a close-up view of the systems and organs discussed during rehabilitation.

breathlessness as well as reduce panic by improving their ventilatory dynamics and pattern. Breathing techniques may help prevent dynamic airway compression, improve respiratory synchrony of abdominal and thoracic musculature, and improve gas exchange by decreasing dynamic hyperinflation, increasing tidal volume, and slowing respiratory rate.[24-26] Teaching paced breathing is useful to enhance the patient's ability to perform activities of daily living with less shortness of breath.[27] Using a pulse oximeter (a form of biofeedback) to demonstrate an increase in oxygen saturation while performing pursed-lip breathing may increase patient use of proper breathing techniques.[28]

Bronchial Hygiene

Bronchial hygiene techniques are appropriate for patients who have considerable difficulty clearing sputum.[29] Bronchial hygiene instruction may include the following:

- Cough techniques[30]
- Postural drainage[31]
- Percussion (manual or mechanically assisted with a vest)
- Vibration
- Positive airway pressure[32]
- Positive expiratory pressure (PEP or flutter valves)[33]
- Autogenic drainage[34]

Having a thorough knowledge of these techniques, and the specific needs of the patient, will enable the pulmonary rehabilitation practitioner

to match the most effective technique(s) to the patient's needs. Patients using inhaled bronchodilators should be instructed in the importance of using their bronchodilator prior to performing bronchial hygiene techniques. If supplemental oxygen is used

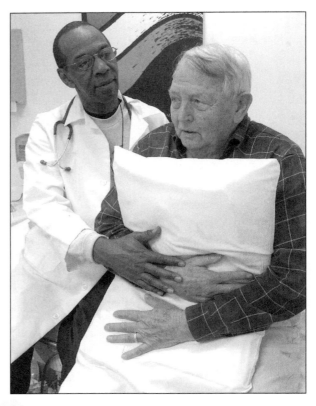

Patients need to be instructed about proper bronchial hygiene, including correct coughing techniques.

during exercise, it may also be necessary during bronchial hygiene techniques. The demonstration of bronchial hygiene techniques is encouraged, and repeated instruction may be necessary.

Medications

Although the primary care or referring physician is responsible for prescribing medications, it is the role of the pulmonary rehabilitation staff to educate the patient regarding these medications. Education in the prescribed dosage, frequency, side effects, interactions, and role of medications in the treatment of respiratory disease is of utmost importance to all patients.[26,35-37] Although the primary emphasis in pulmonary rehabilitation is on respiratory medications (including oxygen), it is also important that the proper use of all of medications be addressed. Patients should understand the importance of maintaining a list of all medications and of telling all health care providers what medications they are taking, including complementary, alternative, and over-the-counter medications. This should reduce the possibility of harmful drug interactions. Medication instruction should be individualized and include a return demonstration of inhaler or spacer use. A major outcome measure of patient responsibility is adherence to the medication regimen.

Exercise Principles

The benefits of exercise for improving patients' functional capacity and activities of daily living are well established (see chapter 4).[38,39] Teaching this information underscores the importance of adherence to the individualized exercise program. To facilitate continued adherence, practitioners should develop a home exercise program for each patient prior to the completion of pulmonary rehabilitation. An exercise log or diary may be developed for patients to self-record their home exercise. The benefits of lifelong exercise should be stressed, and patients should be encouraged to continue in a maintenance exercise program (see appendix B.)

Activities of Daily Living

Independence in activities of daily living is a primary goal for patients with chronic respiratory disease. Patients' individualized treatment plans are established based on the initial assessment. The goal of the treatment plan is to provide patients with the tools necessary to adapt to their limitations and improve their quality of life. The train-

ing sessions may include but are not limited to the following areas:

- Energy conservation[40]
- Work simplification
- Time management techniques
- Panic control
- Relaxation techniques
- Pacing techniques
- Food procurement and preparation
- Leisure activities[41]
- Adaptive equipment
- Sexuality[42]
- Travel considerations[43]
- Community resources
- Vocational retraining

Respiratory Devices and Modalities

Patients with chronic respiratory disease frequently use various types of respiratory therapy modalities and equipment to aid their breathing. The use of specific modalities is based on the patient's disease and individual needs. Reinforcement and additional education and training may be necessary to ensure that patients are correctly using their modalities and are compliant with their physician's prescription. Education and training on respiratory devices and modalities may include the following:

- Metered-dose and dry powder inhalers[44]
- Nebulizers/compressors[45]
- Peak flow meters[46]
- Oxygen delivery systems (concentrators, liquid, compressed gas)[47]
- Oxygen-conserving devices[48]
- Transtracheal oxygen (TTO)[49]
- Inspiratory muscle training[50]
- Positive expiratory pressure[32,33]
- Sleep assessment equipment (oximetry, apnea monitors)
- CPAP and BiPAP
- Suctioning in the home[51]
- Tracheostomy care[52]
- Ventilator management in the home[53,54]

Instruction should include the proper use, care, and cleaning of home respiratory equipment.

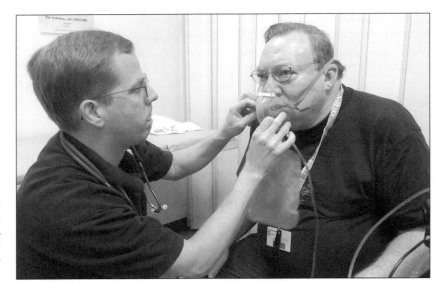

Teaching patients the proper use of breathing equipment is vital to any pulmonary rehabilitation program. Patients must be instructed in how to use and care for their breathing equipment.

Self-Management Strategies Including Smoking Cessation

Self-management strategies for patients with chronic respiratory disease are geared toward slowing the progression and avoiding complications of the disease. The major intervention in reducing the progression of respiratory disease is smoking cessation. Patients must learn to avoid environmental and occupational irritants, especially first- and second-hand cigarette smoke. The respiratory exacerbation is an extremely important factor in morbidity, mortality, and health resource use. Early recognition of signs and symptoms of the respiratory exacerbation and knowledge of when to seek additional medical intervention as well as the importance of discussing with their health care provider the appropriateness of receiving the influenza and/or pneumonia immunization should be included in education and training.[26] Simple techniques such as hand washing and covering the mouth when coughing are often overlooked in instructional sessions. The following is a list of specific topics for discussion with pulmonary rehabilitation participants:

- Smoking cessation[55]
- Hazards of secondhand smoke
- Environmental and occupational irritant avoidance
- When to call your health care provider
- Signs and symptoms of a respiratory infection
- Management strategies for increased symptoms and exacerbations

- Dyspnea management
- Vaccinations (influenza and pneumococcal)

Nutrition

General nutritional principles apply to all patients who have chronic respiratory disease (see chapter 2). The pulmonary patient can fall anywhere along the weight spectrum, from severe nutritional depletion to morbid obesity. Patients should be educated on the reasons for their nutritional abnormalities, such as the increased metabolic cost of breathing resulting in weight loss, or a sedentary lifestyle and oral corticosteroids resulting in weight gain. Instruction should be geared to the individual needs of the patient, as determined on initial and follow-up assessments. Osteoporosis is epidemic in people with chronic lung disease and should be addressed in educational as well as exercise sessions. In some instances, it may be beneficial to refer the patient for intensive dietary counseling. Examples of nutritional topics to cover with patients include the following:

- Reasons and need for weight loss or gain[55-57]
- Adequate fluid intake
- Special diets: sodium restriction, food allergies, cholesterol reduction, reflux diet
- The problem of early satiety
- Size and frequency of meals
- Aerophagia (air swallowing)
- Diabetic training
- Prevention, diagnosis, and treatment of osteopenia or osteoporosis

- Alcohol consumption/restriction
- The potential use of anabolic steroids to treat nutritional depletion
- The complementary roles of diet and exercise as weight loss strategies

Ethical Issues and Advance Directives

Advance directives, including living wills and durable powers of attorney for health care, are underused in the general population. This problem is especially prevalent in the geriatric population. These topics are particularly important to discuss with patients with chronic respiratory disease because of the frequency of respiratory failure and the potential need for mechanical ventilation in this population. Advance directives help to improve communication among the patient, family, and physician should be incorporated into the treatment plan. This plan is derived from patients' understanding of their disease, the ramifications of dialing 9-1-1, the implications of resuscitation in the home, their values and life goals, and the physician's estimation of mortality and morbidity outcomes in certain clinical situations.

If the decision is made to limit medical intervention given by emergency medical services (EMS) providers in nonacute care hospital settings (e.g., the home, a long-term care facility, or during transport to or from a health care facility), specific rules or laws may apply. Information and sample forms of a prehospital medical care directive, as well as a living will and durable power of attorney for health care for use in the hospital setting, are available from a county medical society, hospital association, or local EMS provider. Examples of ethical issues to cover with patients include the following:

- Advance directives[59-61]
- Living wills
- Durable power of attorney for health care
- Prehospital medical care directive
- Ramifications of dialing 9-1-1 for the person with advance directives
- Specific rules or laws that may limit medical intervention outside the acute care setting

Psychosocial Issues

Some patients cope better than others with the emotional aspects of chronic respiratory disease.[62] Group interaction is often successful in helping patients share their coping mechanisms. The staff should provide individualized assistance. Chapter 5 provides additional information on psychosocial intervention strategies. If severe psychosocial issues arise, the patient may warrant a referral for counseling. Some areas of psychosocial intervention that may be discussed are as follows:

- Strategies for coping with lung disease
- Depression management
- Panic control
- Stress reduction
- Relaxation techniques
- Anger control
- Support systems
- Patient–caregiver relationships
- Well spouse issues
- Sexuality
- Modifying addictive behaviors (e.g., nicotine, alcohol, prescribed medication, illegal drugs, etc.)
- Memory improvement skills

Conclusion

Patient education and skills training join assessment, exercise training, and psychosocial support as essential components of pulmonary rehabilitation. Pulmonary rehabilitation education and skills training help the patient and significant other(s) develop a working knowledge of the disease process and foster an appropriate, effective treatment program of collaborative self-management. In general, attainment of educational goals requires a minimum of 20 hours. Patients should be aware of the nature of their disease and its resultant disturbances of function, as well as the purpose and value of each aspect of care. Rehabilitation team members should be sensitive to patients' expectations and work with them to set realistic goals. This will allow patients to take control of their disease, improve their adherence to treatment recommendations, and lessen their fears and anxiety.

Equally as important as the initial educational process is long-term adherence to the principles learned. This can be augmented by offering continuing education opportunities either formally or informally. Support groups that include an educational component or simply reviewing concepts with the patient as they walk on the treadmill can be effective methods for improving compliance with self-management skills.

chapter 4

Exercise Assessment and Training

Exercise intolerance and functional impairment are common consequences of chronic respiratory disease. The benefits of exercise training for improving dyspnea, functional capacity, performance of activities of daily living, and quality of life have been well established.[1] Exercise assessment and training should therefore be essential components of comprehensive pulmonary rehabilitation programs.

Exercise Assessment

Exercise assessment of the patient with chronic pulmonary disease may be used to

- quantify exercise capacity prior to beginning a program,[2,3]
- establish a baseline for outcome documentation,[4]
- assist in formulating an exercise prescription for exercise training,[3,4,5,6]
- detect exercise-induced hypoxemia and aid with dosing supplemental oxygen therapy,[7]
- evaluate nonpulmonary limitations to exercise (e.g., musculoskeletal problems),[2,3]
- help detect underlying cardiac abnormalities,[2,3] and
- screen for exercise-induced bronchospasm.[8]

For most respiratory patients without known or suspected cardiac problems, exercise testing, even to maximum levels, is relatively safe. Contraindications to exercise testing in this setting are thus relatively few. Standard lists of absolute and relative contraindication[3] are concerned primarily with patients with known or suspected cardiovascular abnormalities contraindications (see figure 4.1). One exception may be the individual with primary pulmonary vascular disease with pulmonary hypertension (i.e., primary pulmonary hypertension or chronic thromboembolic pulmonary embolism). In such individuals, some experts advise caution with higher levels of exercise training because of the risk of serious cardiac arrhythmias or even sudden death.

A variety of exercise testing procedures and protocols have been used to evaluate patients in pulmonary rehabilitation programs. No single testing protocol is clearly established as the most

appropriate for all patients and programs. Selection of an appropriate exercise test may depend on

- individual patient status and goals,
- program objectives,
- questions identified in the initial patient assessment (see chapter 2),
- type of exercise training program,
- available laboratory resources, and
- cost.

In the pulmonary patient, formal exercise testing is generally of two types: walk distance test (WDTs) and incremental maximal exercise test (IMETs). WDTs are easier to perform, the results correlate well with functional status, and they can identify the need for supplemental oxygen.[9] In contrast, IMETs are more complex to perform, but they stress the cardiopulmonary system maximally and better define the absolute limits on a patient (including supplemental oxygen needs and the propensity for exercise bronchospasm).[2,8]

Figure 4.1 Contraindications to Exercise Testing

Absolute
- A recent significant change in the resting ECG suggesting significant ischemia, recent myocardial infarction (within 2 days), or other acute cardiac event
- Unstable angina
- Uncontrolled cardiac arrhythmias causing symptoms or hemodynamic compromise
- Severe symptomatic aortic stenosis
- Uncontrolled symptomatic heart failure
- Acute pulmonary embolus or pulmonary infarction
- Acute myocarditis or pericarditis
- Suspected or known dissecting aneurysm
- Acute infections

Relative[†]
- Left main coronary artery stenosis
- Moderate stenotic valvular heart disease
- Electrolyte abnormalities (e.g., hypokalemia, hypomagnesemia)
- Severe arterial hypertension (i.e., systolic BP of >200 mmHg and/or a diastolic BP of >110 mmHg) at rest
- Tachyarrhythmias or bradyarrhythmias
- Hypertrophic cardiomyopathy and other forms of outflow tract obstruction
- Neuromuscular, musculoskeletal, or rheumatoid disorders that are exacerbated by exercise
- High-degree atrioventricular block
- Ventricular aneurysm
- Uncontrolled metabolic disease (e.g., diabetes, thyrotoxicosis, or myxedema)
- Chronic infectious disease (e.g., mononucleosis, hepatitis, AIDS)

† = Relative contraindications can be superseded if benefits outweigh the risks of exercise. In some instances, these individuals can be exercised with caution or using low-level end points, especially if they are asymptomatic at rest.

Reprinted, by permission, from American College of Sports Medicine, 2000, *ACSM's guidelines for exercise testing and prescription*, 6th ed. (Philadelphia, PA: Lippincott, Williams, and Wilkins), 50.

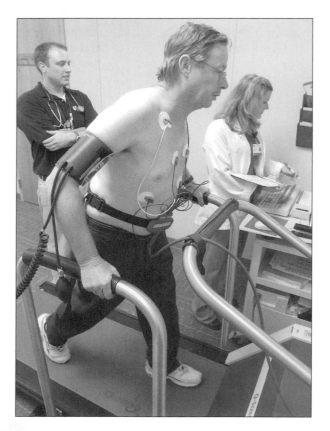

Laboratory tests such as the stress test can be used to assess a patient's physical fitness. Practitioners should determine the fitness level of patients before starting a rehabilitation program.

Walk Distance Tests

WDTs are of two types: timed WDTs and shuttle WDTs. The 6-minute timed WDT is a widely reported outcome measure for pulmonary rehabilitation.[9,10] To obtain valid and reliable results, however, it is essential to standardize the test procedure (e.g., number of tests at baseline, patient instructions, reinforcement during testing, use of supplemental oxygen, and so on).[9]

The 6-minute WDT is performed on a premeasured walking distance such as in a hallway or on a track, not on a treadmill. The patient is instructed to walk as far as possible during the 6-minute time interval. The distance walked (in feet or meters) is recorded as well as the number of times the patient stopped to rest and the total time spent resting. It is also reasonable to periodically monitor pulse oximetry and heart rate. Figure 4.2 shows a sample evaluation form for use in the 6-minute WDT. One can also calculate MET level (one MET is the amount of energy required while the body is at rest) using the distance and time walked during a WDT, and this may be useful information in formulating an initial exercise prescription (see figure 4.3).

Timed Distance Walk Evaluation Form

	Initial 6-minute walk			Discharge 6-minute walk		
	Pre-walk	Walk: #1	#2	Pre-walk	Walk: #1	#2
Total distance (ft)	_____	_____	_____	_____	_____	_____
Inside/outside	_____	_____	_____	_____	_____	_____
# rests	_____	_____	_____	_____	_____	_____
Time of rest (s)	_____	_____	_____	_____	_____	_____
Borg scale	_____	_____	_____	_____	_____	_____
SO_2	_____	_____	_____	_____	_____	_____
F_iO_2	_____	_____	_____	_____	_____	_____
O_2 L/m	_____	_____	_____	_____	_____	_____
BPmax	_____	_____	_____	_____	_____	_____
HRmax	_____	_____	_____	_____	_____	_____
MPH	_____	_____	_____	_____	_____	_____
METs	_____	_____	_____	_____	_____	_____
Patient symptoms (see key)	_____	_____	_____	_____	_____	_____
Supportive devices used (see key)	_____	_____	_____	_____	_____	_____
Other comments:	_____	_____	_____	_____	_____	_____
	_____	_____	_____	_____	_____	_____
	_____	_____	_____	_____	_____	_____
Staff initials:	_____	_____	_____	_____	_____	_____
Date:	_____	_____	_____	_____	_____	_____

Key:

Patient symptoms: chest pain, dizziness, shortness of breath, leg pain, cramps, etc. Supportive walking devices used: walker, cart, wheelchair, cane, etc.

Staff signatures: _____

_____

Figure 4.2 Pulmonary rehabilitation timed distance walk evaluation form.

One MET is the level of energy expenditure at rest or at approximately 3.5 ml/kg/min of oxygen consumption. Activities are expressed as requiring a multiple of this resting requirement. MET levels during walking may be calculated by using the following formula (1 ml/kg/min of oxygen consumption is required for 10 meters/min of walking):

METs = (Baseline MET + walk MET) / Baseline MET

Example: 100 meters walked in a 6-minute walk

METS = (3.5 + (100 meters/6 minutes)
         × (minutes/10 meters)) / 3.5 = 1.47

Figure 4.3 Calculating MET levels from WDTs.

The shuttle WDT measures a symptom-limited walking distance over a marked walking course of usually 10 meters.[11,12,13] It also utilizes an audible pacing timer to incrementally increase pacing frequency (table 4.1), although some use a simpler constant pacing strategy. The subject walks according to the pacing timer frequency until exhaustion. The shuttle WDT is thus more a test of endurance than the timed WDT. Like the timed WDT, however, the primary test result of the shuttle WDT is the total distance walked. Parameters such as heart rate, blood pressure, and pulse oximetry can also be recorded. Shuttle WDTs have been used in both cardiac and pulmonary rehabilitation programs to quantify outcome.[11,12,13] Proponents argue that the shuttle WDT results are less affected by motivation

Table 4.1 Example of Layout and Pacing Algorithm for Shuttle Walk Distance Test

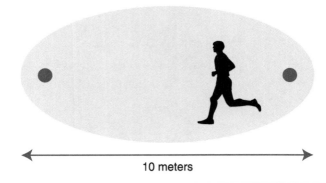

10 meters

Level	Speed m/s	Number of shuttles per level	Distance ambulated at the end of each level (m)
1	0.50	3	30
2	0.67	4	70
3	0.84	5	120
4	1.01	6	180
5	1.18	7	250
6	1.35	8	330
7	1.52	9	420
8	1.69	10	520
9	1.86	11	630
10	2.03	12	750
11	2.20	13	880
12	2.37	14	1020

Reprinted, with permission, from S.J. Singh et al., 1992, "Development of a shuttle walking test of disability in patients with chronic airways obstruction," *Thorax* 47: 1019-1024.

or pacing, correlate better with exercise capacity in patients with chronic lung disease, and may be more sensitive indicators of functional change with rehabilitation and other therapies.[10,11,12,13]

Incremental Maximal Exercise Test

Maximal exercise tolerance is typically measured with an IMET performed on a treadmill or stationary bicycle in a laboratory.[2,3,14] Arm ergometry may be substituted for those patients who are unable to perform lower extremity exercises. The IMET provides either ramped or incremental increases in exercise load (e.g., 15-25 watts/min) until patients reach a symptom-limited maximum. Physiologic responses to this graded exercise are commonly evaluated with ECG monitoring, blood pressure determinations, pulse oximetry, and ratings of perceived symptoms of breathlessness and muscle fatigue. Symptoms can be rated by using the Borg category scale[15] of breathlessness (figure 4.4) or a

visual analog scale (figure 4.5). With the addition of expired gas analysis to the IMET, evaluation of oxygen consumption, carbon dioxide production, and measurement of the anaerobic threshold (when reached) can be performed.[2,3,14] The addition of arterial blood gas analysis allows for the most accurate assessment of arterial oxygenation (i.e., alveolar–arterial oxygen gradient), carbon dioxide levels, dead space/tidal volume ratio (Vd/Vt), and acid–base balance measurements.

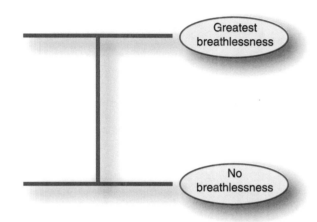

Figure 4.5 Visual analog scale.
Adapted from R.C.B. Aitken, 1969, "Measurement of feelings using visual analogue scales." *Proc R. Soc Med* 62:989-993.

In respiratory patients, two other assessments should also be considered during the IMET. First, dynamic hyperinflation can develop with increasing ventilation; this can be assessed periodically with maximal flow-volume loops.[14] Second, exercise-induced bronchospasm can be assessed by spirometry for up to 30 minutes postexercise.[8] Commonly used criteria to define specific limitations to exercise are given in figure 4.6.

Submaximal Exercise Test

Although less commonly used in pulmonary rehabilitation programs, submaximal, steady-state exercise testing can be performed to assess supplemental oxygen requirements for activities of daily living (ADLs). In this situation the test is conducted at a work rate that approximates those encountered during normal living conditions. A submaximal exercise test may also be conducted with patients with severe pulmonary hypertension or congestive heart failure, for whom maximal stress testing is contraindicated. Symptoms can be rated by using the Borg or visual analog scales.

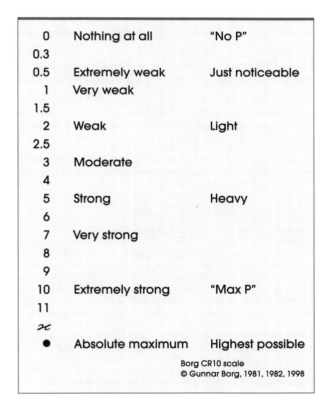

0	Nothing at all	"No P"
0.3		
0.5	Extremely weak	Just noticeable
1	Very weak	
1.5		
2	Weak	Light
2.5		
3	Moderate	
4		
5	Strong	Heavy
6		
7	Very strong	
8		
9		
10	Extremely strong	"Max P"
11		
∞		
●	Absolute maximum	Highest possible

Borg CR10 scale
© Gunnar Borg, 1981, 1982, 1998

Figure 4.4 Category scale of breathlessness, a perceived symptom scale used to rate symptoms of breathlessness and fatigue during exercise testing.
Reprinted, by permission, from G.A. Borg, 1998, *Borg's perceived exertion and pain scales* (Champaign, IL: Human Kinetics), 50.

Figure 4.6 Criteria for Determining Limitations During a Symptom-Limited Incremental Exercise Test

Ventilatory Limits
Max exercise $\dot{V}_E$/MVV > 80%
Rising P_aCO_2
Rising V_D/V_T
Development of dynamic hyperinflation
Development of exercise-induced bronchospasm

Gas Exchange Limits
Falling S_aO_2 or S_pO_2

Cardiovascular Limits
Exercise HR >80% age-predicted max heart rate
Falling blood pressure
Serious dysrhythmias
Cardiac symptoms (e.g., chest pain)
Hypertensive or hypotensive response
Deconditioning

Other Limits
Orthopedic
Peripheral vascular
Musculoskeletal
Metabolic
Motivational or psychological

Exercise Assessment Equipment

The following lists detail equipment you will need to conduct WDTs and IMEs.

WDTs

- A measured walking distance with minimal traffic used for timed distance walk tests (at least 100 feet for timed WDTs or 10 meters for shuttle WDTs)
- Manual blood pressure measurement equipment
- Stethoscope
- Cutaneous pulse oximeter
- Supplemental oxygen source
- Stopwatch
- Borg scale chart
- Walker, cart, or wheelchair
- Emergency plan and supplies (refer to your hospital's or facility's policy; should include bronchodilators)
- Audible walking pacer (shuttle WDTs)

- Test-site personnel trained in basic life support techniques

Additional equipment for IME tests

- Calibrated cycle ergometer or motorized treadmill
- Equipment to monitor EKG during exercise testing
- Defibrillator and crash cart
- Access to a laboratory for arterial blood gas analysis
- Equipment for expired gas analysis to measure VO_2 (oxygen uptake), VCO_2 (carbon dioxide elimination), minute ventilation, and various derived variables
- Spirometry equipment for use in assessing dynamic hyperinflation and exercise-induced bronchospasm

Functional Performance Assessment

In addition to formal exercise testing, patients should also be assessed by questioning and exams regarding functional performance status. This should include evaluation of respiratory muscle function (e.g., diaphragmatic excursion, thoracoabdominal synchrony) as well as any orthopedic limitations or other musculoskeletal contraindications to exercise. Figure 4.7 outlines some of the important considerations in this assessment.[16]

Musculoskeletal problems can be especially prominent in the older pulmonary rehabilitation

---

Figure 4.7 Functional Status Assessment Considerations

Muscle strength and endurance
Joint pains, limited range of motion, or both
Oxygen needs
Subjective endurance and work tolerance
Dyspnea
Lack of understanding of fitness and exercise
Fear of exertion
Inability to pace activities
Balance abnormalities
Gait instability
Pain levels and locations

---

population. It is important to make a thorough assessment of the patient's baseline levels of strength, range of motion, posture, orthopedic limitations, and simple activities of ADL movements (e.g., transfers such as sitting to standing and lying to standing).[16,17]

Exercise Training

Many factors must be considered when selecting an exercise plan for persons with respiratory disease. The pulmonary rehabilitation clinician should be aware of these factors regarding exercise for this population.

Mechanisms of Exercise Intolerance in Chronic Respiratory Disease

Respiratory and nonrespiratory factors, alone or in combination, can significantly decrease the exercise tolerance of persons with chronic lung disease (see figure 4.6).[18,19,20,21,22,23,24,25] Although cardiopulmonary factors are generally considered the most important,[20,22,24,25] skeletal muscle dysfunction

has been increasingly recognized as a key factor that contributes to exercise intolerance.[26,27] Indeed, the perception of leg effort or discomfort is the main symptom that limits exercise in 40% to 45% of patients with COPD.[25,26] Skeletal muscle dysfunction in COPD is characterized by reductions in muscle mass and strength;[28,29] atrophy of slow-twitch, oxidative endurance muscle fibers;[30,31,32] reductions in fiber capillarization;[33] oxidative enzyme capacity;[34,35,36] and muscle endurance.[27,37,38] Both resting and exercise muscle metabolism are impaired,[27,35,39,40] and patients experience lower exercise tolerance[41,42] and develop lactic acidosis at lower exercise workloads than healthy persons.[26,43] Systemic inflammation, nutritional impairment, aging, reactive oxygen species, low anabolic hormone levels, corticosteroid-related myopathy, and hypoxia can all contribute to the skeletal muscle dysfunction in COPD.[27,44,45]

Complicating all of these disease effects is deconditioning. This is a consequence of the patient assuming a more sedentary lifestyle to avoid the unpleasant sensation of dyspnea. This inactivity in turn leads to further deconditioning and increased exertional dyspnea creating the "dyspnea spiral" depicted in figure 4.8.

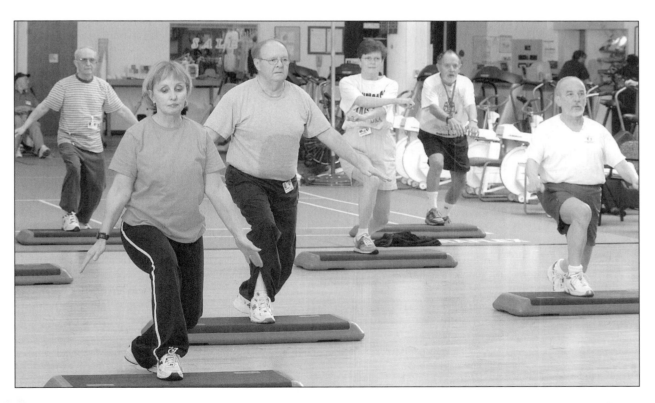

Exercise can help counter the muscular effects of pulmonary diseases. Group exercise can motivate patients.

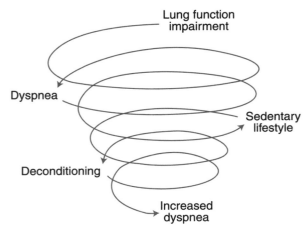

Figure 4.8 Dyspnea spiral.

Reprinted, by permission, from C. Prefaunt, A. Varray, and G. Vallet, 1995, "Pathophysiological basis of exercise training in patients with chronic obstructive lung disease," *European Respiratory Review* 5 (25): 27-32.

Rationale for Exercise Training in Chronic Lung Disease

Patients with chronic lung disease are capable of aerobic conditioning if their disease process does not prevent them from achieving training levels of exercise. Thus, patients able to achieve high exercise heart rates without gas exchange, ventilatory, or other developing limitations should be expected to derive significant benefit from formal exercise training.[46,47,48] Optimizing oxygenation and bronchodilation will help achieve these goals. The presence of skeletal muscle dysfunction provides further rationale for exercise training for patients with COPD, even in the presence of significant cardiopulmonary limitations imposed by the presence of irreversible derangements of lung structure or function. A supervised exercise program can also address other factors limiting exercise in these patients such as fear of dyspnea, psychological issues, and musculoskeletal factors. Taken together, all of these effects of a formal supervised exercise program in chronic lung disease can all help reverse the downward dyspnea spiral of figure 4.8 and improve function.[1,4,6,46,49,52,53] Indeed, the evidence base supporting the functional benefits of exercise training in COPD is among the strongest in pulmonary medicine.[1,50,51,52,53,54,55] Because of this, exercise training is a necessary component of comprehensive pulmonary rehabilitation.

Exercise Duration, Frequency, Mode, and Intensity

Exercise training in pulmonary rehabilitation should encompass both lower and upper extremity endurance training, strength training, and possibly respiratory muscle training. Duration, frequency, mode, and intensity of exercise should be included in the patient's individualized exercise prescription based on disease severity, degree of conditioning, and initial exercise test data. Various guidelines for exercise training have been suggested.[3,4,48] Aerobic endurance training may be performed at high or low intensity. High intensity training (e.g., at 60% to 80% Wmax) must be undertaken to gain physiologic improvements in aerobic fitness such as increased $\dot{V}O_2max$, delayed anaerobic threshold, decreased HR for a given VO_2, increased oxidative enzyme capacity, and capillarization of muscle following training.[6,56,57,58,59,60] Such improvements can result in lower ventilatory requirements for a given exercise task, as well as more efficient patterns of breathing with reduced dead space ventilation (due to increased tidal volume and decreased respiratory rate).[61] These gains are associated with significant gains in exercise endurance.[6] However, not all patients can tolerate sustained high intensity exercise at the outset of training. Patients who exercise at the maximum intensity tolerated can, however, achieve gains in the maximum intensity tolerated over time.[62] Interval training, alternating periods of high versus low intensity exercise, or rest is an effective training option for persons who cannot sustain extended continuous periods of high intensity exercise.[63,64]

It is important to note that it is not absolutely necessary to achieve improvement in physical parameters of aerobic fitness to achieve gains in exercise tolerance. This is important, since high intensity exercise may lead to a greater degree of dyspnea and leg fatigue and therefore may be less likely to be incorporated into patients' routine lifestyles. Moreover, it has not been proven conclusively that achievement of physiologic gains in aerobic fitness leads to better improvements in day-to-day functional capacity than does lower intensity exercise not leading to these training effects. Lower intensity aerobic exercise training also leads to significant improvements in exercise (treadmill, walking, cycling, and so on) endurance, even in the absence of measured gains in aerobic fitness.[53,60,65,66,67] Furthermore, transcutaneous neuromuscular electrical stimulation can improve lower extremity muscle strength and exercise endurance even in the absence of traditional cardiovascular exercise training,[68,69] and is an option for patients with very severe diseases who are unable or unwilling to participate in a conventional exercise training program. Lower intensity exercise also leads to smaller improvements in dyspnea scores and QOL[1,49] in the absence of post-training physiologic changes. Thus, mechanisms other than cardiovascular conditioning must be operative.

The frequency and duration of the supervised exercise component during a pulmonary rehabilitation program may vary from 3 to 5 times per week, 30 to 90 minutes per session, and over a period of 4 to 12 weeks. Many different modes of exercise training have been used successfully with pulmonary patients, including walking (e.g., treadmill; track; supported walking via walker, cart, or wheelchair), cycling, stationary bicycling, arm ergometry, arm lifting exercises with or without weights, step exercise, rowing, water exercises, swimming, modified aerobic dance, and seated aerobics. Warm-up and cool-down periods must be included in each exercise session. Warm-up exercise allows for gradual increases in heart rate, blood pressure, ventilation, and blood flow to the exercising muscles. Cool-down reduces the risk of arrhythmias, orthostatic hypotension, syncopal episodes, and bronchospasm. Because exercise training is in many ways a tool to help patients learn to cope with the frightening and disabling sensation of breathlessness that often limits their exercise capacity, almost any type of exercise that the patient enjoys or is willing to do can be helpful.

In exercising patients with chronic lung disease, it is important to evaluate and periodically monitor oxyhemoglobin saturation (with cutaneous oximetry or arterial blood gas) with exercise to determine the need for supplemental oxygen. In particular, the arterial oxygen levels of patients with chronic lung disease change with exercise in an unpredictable fashion and cannot be reliably predicted by any measurement made at rest.[7] In general, it is recommended that cutaneous oximetry estimates of oxyhemoglobin saturation be maintained at a level greater than 90% SaO_2 during exercise.[70,71] Cutaneous oximetry only estimates true arterial oxygen saturation within about ± 3% to 5% accuracy (and it tends to overestimate true saturation). Supplemental oxygen therapy, therefore, should be available in the rehabilitation setting for those patients who exhibit a hypoxemic response to exercise. Interestingly, a recent report has suggested that supplemental O_2 might also improve exercise training in COPD patients who do *not* have significant desaturation.[72] The mechanisms underlying this benefit are not clear but might involve decreased carotid body stimulation and reduced pulmonary vascular resistance.

Previously unrecognized exercise-induced oxygen desaturation should be reported to the patient's physician so that consideration can be given to initiate oxygen prescription if needed.

Pulse delivery of oxygen via electronic demand device may not provide adequate oxygen saturation for some patients. Instead, continuous flow delivery of oxygen may be required. Patients should ultimately be tested during the maximal intensity level exercise they may undertake, using the type of portable oxygen system they will use outside the program.

Bronchodilator therapy is also important to optimize during an exercise program. This includes not only assuring that the maintenance regimen is correct, but also that needs for preexercise treatment are addressed. Bronchodilators should also be part of any emergency cart in the exercise area.

Specific Techniques for Upper and Lower Extremity Training

It is most beneficial to direct exercise training to those muscles involved in ADLs. This typically includes training the muscles of both the lower and upper extremities.

Lower extremity training involves large muscle groups; this modality can improve ambulatory stamina, balance, and performance in ADLs.[3] Types of lower extremity training include the following:

- Walking
- Stationary cycling
- Bicycling
- Stair climbing
- Swimming

Aerobic training of the lower extremities improves exercise tolerance of patients with COPD.[1,49,50,65] Randomized controlled trials have demonstrated that lower extremity training of several types increases exercise endurance, and to a lesser extent, maximal work rate.[1,49,50,51,73] Increases of up to 80 meters (10% to 25%) in walk distance,[50,55,73,74,75,76] 10 minutes in treadmill endurance,[53,77] 5 minutes in cycle ergometer time at submaximal workloads,[6,50,61,78] and up to a 36% increase in maximum workload[61] have been reported following 6 to 12 weeks of training. Benefits of training may last up to two years.[79]

Exercise training of the arms is also beneficial. Patients with moderate to severe COPD, especially those with mechanical disadvantage of the diaphragm due to lung hyperinflation, have difficulty performing ADLs that involve use of the upper extremities. Arm elevation is associated with high metabolic and ventilatory demand,[80,81] and activities involving the arms can lead to irregular or dyssynchronous breathing.[82,83] Such alterations in breathing pattern may occur due to derecruitment of accessory respiratory muscles away from their work as muscles of inspiration contributing to arm activity.[83,84,85] In contrast to the lower extremities, intolerance of exercise involving the upper extremities for persons with COPD likely relates more to these altered patterns of muscle utilization and less to physiologic derangements in skeletal muscle.[29,86,87]

Benefits of upper extremity training in COPD include improved arm muscle endurance[88] and strength,[89] reduced metabolic demand associated with arm exercise,[90] and increased sense of well-being.[88,89,90] In general, benefits of upper extremity training are task-specific, that is, noted in performance of the types of tasks for which the muscle groups were trained.[91,92] Upper extremity training is recommended in conjunction with lower extremity training as a routine component of pulmonary rehabilitation.[1,49]

Strength Training

In addition to endurance training, strength training is beneficial for patients with chronic lung disease. Weight lifting may lead to improvements in muscle strength, increased exercise endurance, and fewer symptoms during ADLs.[5,89,91,93,94] Examples of strength training modalities include the following:

- Hand and ankle weights
- Free weights
- Circuit resistance

A recommended approach for strength training prescription has been reviewed.[95] The relative advantages and disadvantages of high- versus low-intensity strength training for persons with COPD are as yet unknown. Safety and prevention of muscle tears is of crucial importance, especially for persons on chronic steroid therapy who may be at risk of muscle or tendon rupture when exposed to high intensity loads. The combination of strength plus aerobic fitness training leads to gains in both strength and endurance.[96,97,98] Although there is no clear synergistic effect from combining these forms of training,[63,95] the combined training approach may lead to improved exercise tolerance for a greater variety of tasks, which may in turn translate into improved performance of ADLs. Since the combination approach is also safe, it is the recommended approach for training patients in the context of pulmonary rehabilitation.

Posture and Body Mechanics

Along with strengthening the upper and lower extremities, various exercises to develop and maintain proper posture and good body symmetry should also be incorporated into a rehabilitation program. A lack of flexibility in particular muscle groups and imbalance in the muscular development of others can result in poor posture. The common postural deficit of rounded shoulders may be due to a lack of muscular endurance in the scapular girdle abductors (i.e., middle trapezius and rhomboids) with a concomitant inflexibility in the

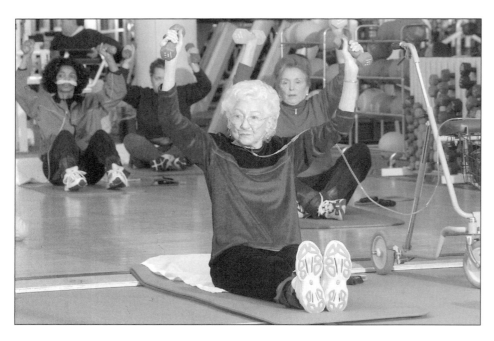

Lightweight training improves a patient's ability to complete everyday tasks such as personal grooming and carrying groceries.

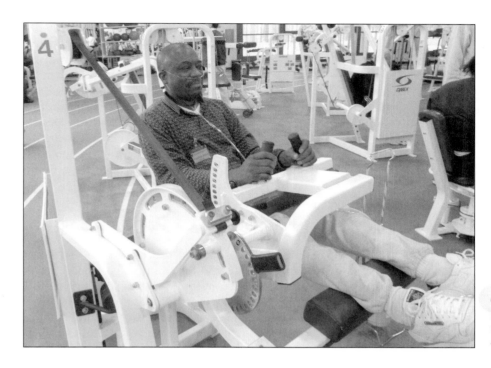

Circuit resistance training helps patients improve muscle strength and exercise endurance.

pectoral muscles of the frontal chest area.[99] Focusing on strengthening the former muscle groups and increasing flexibility in the latter may aid in proper postural formation resulting in improved respiratory mechanics. Incorporating flexibility exercises with a goal to increase range of motion is an integral component of the exercise program. The use of multiple training modalities incorporating flexion and extension exercises is recommended to ensure good posture and proper body mechanics and to minimize joint and muscle injury.

Respiratory Muscle Training

With any exercise, respiratory muscle activity increases and thus the respiratory muscles are exercised. Whether more specific inspiratory muscle activity using resistive breathing devices adds to this is controversial. Some suggest that resistance breathing can lead to an increase in respiratory muscle strength and endurance, as well as a reduction in dyspnea.[100,101,102,103] It has not been established whether this results in an

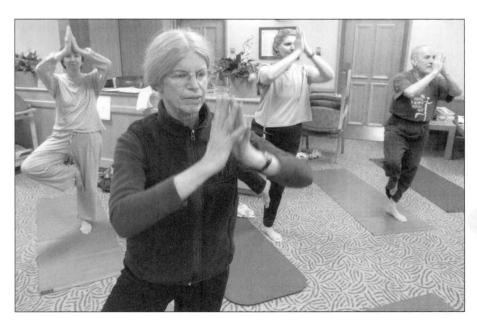

Maintaining flexibility and good posture are important components of a rehabilitation program. Exercises such as yoga help patients maintain needed flexibility and good posture.

improved functional status or exercise capacity for the patient.[104,105]

Types of respiratory muscle training include flow resistive training (breathing through a progressively smaller orifice), threshold loading training (a present inspiratory pressure, usually at some fraction of the maximal inspiratory pressure, is required), and isocapneic hyperventilation.[106] Suggested guidelines for employing resistive inspiratory muscle training include a frequency of four to five days a week; intensities of 30% to 35% of $P_i$max (maximal inspiratory pressure measured at the mouth); and a duration of one 30-minute session per day or two 15-minute sessions[3,17] over at least two to six months. Respiratory muscle training may be considered for patients with known respiratory muscle weakness (e.g., due to cachexia or corticosteroid use) or persons who remain symptomatic with dyspnea and exercise limitation despite peripheral muscle endurance and strength training.[1,49]

Choosing the Site for Exercise Training

Effective exercise training can be undertaken in inpatient, outpatient, and home-based settings. The benefits of training relate to the type and components of the training, rather than the site of training. Outpatient hospital- or office-based training is appropriate for persons with stable moderate to severe diseases who are able to live independently at home and travel to the pulmonary rehabilitation program. Inpatient pulmonary rehabilitation is appropriate for persons with greater severity of illness or functional disability who require 24-hour nursing care, close medical monitoring, or who are unable to perform ADLs and live independently. Inpatient pulmonary rehabilitation is also a setting in which patients undergoing chronic weaning from mechanical ventilation can concomitantly undergo general exercise training and persons can be trained in the care and management of a tracheostomy and home ventilator. Training at home may be appropriate for persons who are unable to leave the home or whose handicaps lead to dependence on assistive devices that preclude the patient from undergoing rehabilitation elsewhere.[107,108]

Patients participating in a formal outpatient rehabilitation program should also be provided with a home exercise prescription, which will encourage them to engage in a continuum of physical activities outside the formal program setting. The home exercise prescription can be developed and begun early in the rehabilitation program, allowing the patient to gain confidence in independent exercise while in the home setting. Usually patients are expected to exercise regularly at home during the program. These unsupervised sessions may be monitored through exercise diaries, which can be reviewed during the supervised exercise sessions. Home exercise also aids the rehabilitation staff in adjusting the exercise prescription and addressing new problems that may arise. This exercise prescription can then be revised for a home maintenance program. Figure 4.9 is a sample form for a home exercise prescription.

Emergency Procedures

Appropriate emergency procedures and supplies must be available in the pulmonary rehabilitation exercise and patient training areas. All staff should be familiar with these emergency procedures. Minimum emergency equipment should include an oxygen source and delivery apparatus, resuscitation mask, first-aid supplies, and bronchodilator medications. In addition, personnel who work with pulmonary patients should be familiar with panic control techniques. In the patient with acute dyspnea, the following are recommended:

- Have the patient stop the activity and assume a comfortable breathing position.
- Encourage the patient to use pursed-lip breathing and relaxation techniques.
- Use bronchodilator medication, if indicated.
- Monitor oxygen saturation.
- Assess cardiovascular status with pulse and BP.
- Administer supplemental oxygen, if indicated.

Conclusion

The importance of an exercise training program cannot be overemphasized. But before a safe exercise program can be provided, a thorough assessment needs to be done to evaluate exercise tolerance, formulate an appropriate exercise training prescription, detect exercise-induced hypoxemia or bronchospasm, and detect occult cardiac or other nonpulmonary limitations to exercise. The benefits of exercise training are well documented. They include increased tolerance for dyspnea, improved appetite, increased physical capability, and improved quality of life. Exercise is one of the essential components of a comprehensive pulmonary rehabilitation program.

Pulmonary Rehabilitation Home Exercise Prescription

Name: _____

The following instructions have been established based on your exercise performance in the pulmonary rehabilitation program. If there is a change in your condition, the instructions may need to be revised.

If you develop chest pain, severe shortness of breath (more than is usually associated with these exercises), or lightheadedness, or feel as if you are about to pass out—stop the exercise and consult your doctor.

If you are having a flare-up of your lung condition, you should not exercise on that day and you should check with your doctor.

When Exercising, REMEMBER:

   A. Use your bronchodilator inhaler or aerosol treatment within 2 hours before you begin to exercise.

   B. Monitor your breathing level and heart rate.

   C. Do pursed-lip breathing.

During Exercise:

   A. On a scale of 0 to 10 (Borg scale), exercise at a maximum breathing level of _____. If you are able to talk, you are OK.

   B. Your target heart rate (THR) is _____ beats/min. Try to stay within your THR. If you are above your THR, do not stop exercising abruptly. Slowly decrease the intensity of the exercise (e.g., walking, biking) until you bring your heart rate down.

   C. If oxygen is prescribed during exercise training, use at _____ L/min.

Types of Exercise:

   1. **Warm-ups**

      Calisthenics: _____ minutes

      Stretching: _____ minutes

      Frequency: _____ daily, _____ ×/week

   2. **Walking/running**

      May also try to walk/run _____ distance in _____ minutes

      Frequency: _____ ×/week

   3. **Supported walking:** _____ minutes (pushing a cart or wheelchair) _____ distance

   4. **Treadmill**

      Speed: _____ miles/hour Duration: _____ minutes Grade of elevation: _____%

      Frequency: _____ ×/week

   5. **Stationary bicycle**

      Speed: _____ miles/hour Duration: _____ minutes Work: _____ watts

      Frequency: _____ ×/week

   6. **Respiratory muscle training**

      Threshold trainer set at _____ cmH_2O Should be done for _____ minutes/day

      Frequency: _____ daily, _____ ×/week

   7. **Strength training**

      Hand weights: _____ sets of _____ repetitions _____ pounds to be used as directed

      Leg weights: _____ sets of _____ repetitions _____ pounds to be used as directed

      Frequency: _____ ×/week

   8. **Abdominal exercises:**

      _____ sets of _____ repetitions Frequency: _____ daily, _____ ×/week

(continued)

Figure 4.9 Sample home pulmonary rehabilitation exercise prescription.

Adapted from Mt. Diablo Medical Center Pulmonary Rehabilitation Program Home Exercise Form, Mt. Diablo Medical Center, Concord, CA, and Temple University Hospital Pulmonary Rehabilitation Program Home Exercise Form, Temple University Hospital, Philadelphia, PA.

9. **Back exercises**

_____ sets of _____ repetitions Frequency: _____ daily, _____ ×/week

10. **Other**

_____

_____

11. **Cool-down exercises**

Lower extremity: _____ minutes

Upper extremity: _____ minutes

Calisthenics: _____ minutes

Stretching: _____ minutes

Frequency: _____ daily, _____ ×/week

12. **Diaphragmatic breathing**

With a _____ pound weight while lying down. Practice your relaxation exercises at this time, for 15 minutes, three to five times/week.

Comments: Do your exercises during the time of day that is best for you. Plan enough time for you to do the exercises without hurrying. Do what you are able to do.

_____

_____

_____

Pulmonary rehabilitation staff: _____ Date: _____

Figure 4.9 *(continued)*

chapter 5

Psychosocial Assessment and Intervention

The courage with which so many patients confront the enormous challenges associated with chronic respiratory disease is truly remarkable. Indeed, the capacity of patients to successfully adapt to these challenges is a major determinant of their quality of life. Although the ways people cope with chronic respiratory disease vary considerably, there are some typical adjustment patterns as well as psychological profiles of which practitioners should be aware. Psychosocial services provided within the pulmonary rehabilitation setting can facilitate the adjustment process by encouraging adaptive thoughts and behaviors, helping patients to reduce negative emotions, and providing a socially supportive environment.

Adjustment Process

In the early stages of chronic respiratory disease, patients and significant others are often unaware of, or deny, the existence and seriousness of the disease. The slow, insidious decline in normal physiological and psychological functioning is often blamed on aging and lack of exercise. The person may cope for many years with cough, sputum production, shortness of breath, and fatigue before an acute exacerbation or pneumonia requires hospitalization. Although characterized by exacerbations and remissions, the disease trajectory is often one of a slowly progressive downward course. The resulting alterations in activity inevitably lead to changes in role, lifestyle, work status, and social and family relationships.

Unlike those of other major diseases, the disabling effects and progression of chronic respiratory disease are not readily visible to the public. This may facilitate for patients to deny the relationship between pulmonary symptoms and past or present behavior, particularly their smoking history. Indeed, even as the disease progresses, evidence suggests that people with chronic respiratory disease are especially adept at suppressing emotions and concerns related to their illness.[1] Although suppressing one's emotions may be adaptive in reducing anxiety levels, denial increases the risk of patient nonadherence with recommended medical interventions and changes in lifestyle.

As the disease progresses, many patients experience fear and anxiety[2] in anticipation of, and in association with, episodes of dyspnea.[3] Conversely, the heightened physiological arousal associated with anxiety can precipitate and exacerbate dyspnea. Therefore, it is not surprising that an anxiety/dyspnea circle may develop and may contribute to inactivity and overall disability in the patient with chronic respiratory disease (see figure 5.1).

Patients' frustration with their poor health and their inability to participate in many simple activities can also present in the form of irritability, pessimism, and a hostile attitude toward others. In many, COPD produces an overall feeling of a loss of self

through loss of roles, identity, and self-esteem. The perceived lack of sympathy for a disease viewed as incurable or self-inflicted is a major reason for this loss of self-esteem.[4] Patients with COPD have

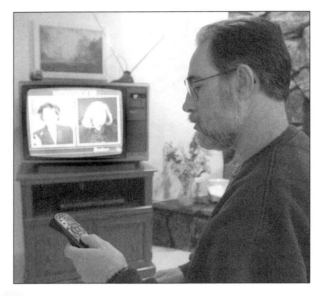

Poor health keeps many patients from doing any type of activity, which can worsen a pulmonary problem. This inactivity can increase feelings of frustration, irritability, and low self-esteem.

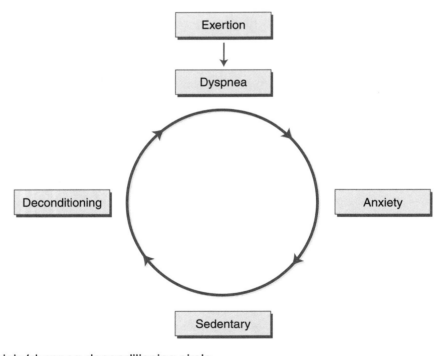

Figure 5.1 Anxiety/dyspnea deconditioning circle.

Adapted, by permission, from L. Hilling and J. Smith, 1995, Pulmonary rehabilitation. In *Cardiopulmonary physical therapy*, 3d ed., edited by S. Irwin and J.S. Tecklin (St. Louis: Mosby).

been reported by relatives to have higher levels of belligerence, negativism, helplessness, withdrawal, psychopathology, nervousness, and confusion than older adults from the general population.[5]

In the later stages of disease, patients may develop a variety of psychosocial symptoms reflecting the progressive feelings of hopelessness and inability to cope with the disease process. Depression is common in patients with moderate to severe COPD,[6,7] with prevalence rates ranging from 7% to 42%.[8] The signs and symptoms of depression include the following:[9]

- Dysphoria (sadness)
- Hopelessness
- Insomnia
- Loss of appetite
- Decreased libido
- Anhedonia (decreased pleasure in activities)
- Decreased energy
- Loss of concentration leading to poor memory
- Suicidal thoughts, particularly a sense of not caring to go on

As in the case of anxiety and dyspnea, a circle of dysfunction may develop in which the loss of energy and desire to participate in physical activity may also contribute to deconditioning and progressive disability. The tendency for depressed patients to withdraw from social interactions outside of the immediate family can further serve to increase feelings of isolation and depression for both patients and their primary caregivers. In contrast, patients may develop even greater dependency on one or more family members for their day-to-day care, which often leads to considerable interpersonal conflict as the patient's needs increase. In addition, sexual activity is often limited by depression, physical limitations, and the development of sustained sexual dysfunction.

As noted previously, mild to moderate neuropsychological impairments may exist as a result of depression as well as hypoxemia, hypercarbia, or both. Such deficits generally involve difficulty in concentrating, poor memory, and problems with general cognitive abilities. Patients experiencing such impairment may have difficulty in solving common problems involved in daily activities, miss office or clinic appointments, and fail to adhere to the medical plan.

Patients with a history of preexisting mental health disorders can be expected to have the greatest difficulty adjusting to the chronic disease process. Particularly noteworthy is the presence of major depressive or anxiety disorders, previous adjustment disorder, personality disorder, alcohol or drug abuse, or a history of psychosis.

As with other chronic illnesses, successful adaptation is often characterized by an active, engaging coping style with a positive, yet realistic, outlook on the future. Psychosocial assets that help those with a chronic illness to cope more effectively include the following:[10]

- A vital interest in life (optimism)
- Adequate financial resources and housing
- Social support
- The ability to cope with modifications in the environment
- Freedom from being overly sensitive
- Congeniality
- Flexibility
- Reliability
- A sense of good judgment

Although some patients may find denying some aspects of their illness helpful, those who use denial or passive acceptance to cope with their illness or treatment requirements often do poorly. A tendency to be preoccupied with somatic symptoms (hypochondriasis) can also limit progress. It is also not surprising that in their efforts to "cope," some patients may self-medicate with alcohol, overuse prescription medications, and maintain other self-destructive behaviors such as cigarette smoking.

An outline of medical and psychosocial stressors experienced by the patient with chronic respiratory disease is presented in figure 5.2. The clinician should also be aware that the patient's spouse or primary caregiver may also be under considerable stress. Though they may be deeply concerned about and dedicated to the patient's welfare, they are often emotionally and physically drained by the daily demands of their caregiving role. This may be particularly evident if caregivers perceive that the patient has become overly dependent on them.

Psychosocial Assessment

Just as exercise capacity and functional abilities are evaluated and to complete the full evaluative process, the psychosocial status of the new

> **Figure 5.2** Medical and Psychosocial Stressors Associated With Chronic Pulmonary Disease
>
> **Medical**
>
> - Dyspnea, fatigue
> - Medication side effects
> - Changes in physique as a result of disease process, medications, deconditioning, and aging
> - Physical limitations imposed by disease (e.g., decreased ability to perform activities of daily living) and treatments (e.g., traveling with oxygen)
> - Loss of cognitive functioning (concentration and memory)
> - Comorbidity (e.g., heart disease, arthritis, cataracts)
> - Sleep deprivation (e.g., from depression, hypoxemia)
> - Surgical complications
>
> **Psychosocial**
>
> - Sense of impending mortality (both of self and other patients they have met in the program)
> - Change in social roles
> - Sexual dysfunction
> - Family demands and reactions from others
> - Public embarrassment (e.g., as a result of oxygen use)
> - Loss of job or income
> - Self-blaming
> - Lack of visible signs of illness
> - Major life events and other significant ongoing stressors (e.g., financial difficulties, comorbidity, legal concerns, role reversal)

pulmonary rehabilitation patient must be assessed by the pulmonary rehabilitation team.

Clinical Assessment

The psychosocial component of the interview and assessment process by an experienced and designated member of the pulmonary rehabilitation team is critical to the success of pulmonary rehabilitation. The time and interest of the interviewer is the cornerstone on which the essential trust relationship between practitioner and patient is built. The interview should allow adequate time for patients to openly express concerns about the psychosocial adjustment to their disease. Screening questionnaires are available to complement the psychosocial information obtained by interview (see appendix A).

Although moderate levels of anxiety or depression may be addressed in the pulmonary rehabilitation program, patients identified as having significant psychosocial disturbances should be referred to an appropriate mental health practitioner, such as a clinical social worker, psychiatric nurse, psychologist, chaplain, or psychiatrist, prior to the start of the program. Significant disturbances include dysfunction in terms of the patient's ability to carry out activities of daily living, high scores in psychometric testing, or acknowledgment by the patient or a support person.

Practitioners are generally most effective in gathering quality assessment information through a combination of unstructured (open-ended questions) and structured (close-ended questions) interviewing formats. The practitioner can convey genuine empathy for the patient's welfare through the use of active listening skills such as the following:

- Making appropriate eye contact
- Paraphrasing and summarizing patients' statements
- Asking questions to clarify important issues
- Employing gentle, nonjudgmental confrontation regarding incongruence between patient statements and behaviors

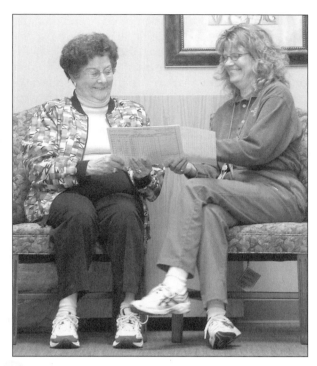

Patients and practitioners must have a strong relationship of trust. Taking the time to get to know your patients and their individual needs is vital.

Interview questions should cover the following areas:

- Perception of quality of life and ability to adjust to the disease.
- Screening for psychopathology (i.e., depression, anxiety).
- Screening for significant neuropsychological impairment (e.g., memory, attention/concentration, and problem-solving abilities during daily activities). If cognitive impairment is suspected from the interview, a specific tool such as the Mini-Mental Status Exam can be administered.

To determine what motivates the patient, the interviewer may ask questions such as the following:

- On a scale of 1 to 10, how ready are you to make a lifestyle change now?
- Who or what inspired you to start pulmonary rehabilitation?
- What do you see as the barriers to successfully completing the program?
- What do you see as the benefits to successfully completing the program?

To determine the potential factors affecting adherence, the interviewer may ask the following:

- What problems are you encountering with taking medication? (Discuss side effects, cost, satisfaction with your primary care physician, forgetting, difficulty with medication delivery systems, and family stressors.)
- Do you believe the medications and treatments are the best ones for your lung problem?
- When you feel better or worse, do you sometimes stop taking your medication?

To learn about the patient's smoking behavior, the interviewer may ask the following:

- Are you currently smoking? If so, are you ready to set a quit date?
- When did you quit? For how long and how much did you smoke?
- How did you handle relapses?
- Are you addicted to other tobacco products, drugs, or alcohol?

To learn about the patient's current level of sexual function, the interviewer may ask the following:

- What are your recent patterns of sexual activity? How have breathing problems affected your sex life?
- What are your current fears and concerns (e.g., shortness of breath during sexual activity, development of impotence)?
- Do you have a sexual partner?
- What is your partner's reaction to the disease and its effect on mutual sexual function?
- What factors other than illness may be affecting your sexual functioning (e.g., age, medications, substance abuse, menopause, partner's health and emotional state)?

Practitioners may wish to interview significant caregivers to gain a second perspective on the patient's medical history and to explore more fully issues related to dependency, interpersonal conflict, and intimacy. Such interviews should be conducted with the patient's consent and performed in a sensitive manner so as not to offend either the patient or the caregiver. Common feelings and concerns that are expressed in this component of the evaluation include guilt, anger, resentment, abandonment, fears, anxieties, helplessness, isolation, grief, pity, sadness, stress, poor sleep, poor marital relations, and failing health of the spouse or caretaker.[11]

All health team members who assess the patient should participate in the discussion of potential psychosocial issues. In particular, identifying and treating associated depression could make a significant difference in the patient's quality of life because depressive symptoms may contribute more to functional disability, poor health perception, and poor well-being than the chronic medical condition itself.[12] In fact, several studies indicate that pharmacotherapy to treat depression or anxiety in patients with COPD improves functional capacity.[12,13] Stabilization of an acute psychiatric problem is essential before beginning pulmonary rehabilitation to ensure a successful experience for the individual and for the treatment team as a whole.

Special Considerations for Psychosocial Assessment

There are several areas of assessment that you must complete in order to mold your interventions more accurately for each individual patient.

Motivation

Motivation has been defined as the "belief that change is worthwhile."[14] It is one of the most important of the psychosocial elements affecting participation in pulmonary rehabilitation, and is influenced by multiple internal and external factors. The Health Belief Model (HBM) is a well-established theoretical framework that proposes the likelihood of a person to follow a recommended health action.[15] It outlines three components that contribute to the patient's motivation: (1) a cue to action, (2) perceived severity of the health condition (or the patient's susceptibility to it), and (3) perceived benefits of and barriers to the behavior change.

Most patients who enter pulmonary rehabilitation have been exposed to a cue to action, such as a physician diagnosing them with COPD, a recent hospitalization, or a spouse who has become concerned about the patient's health. This provides an incentive to many who might not take the initiative to enter pulmonary rehabilitation.

Patients who perceive their illness to be relatively severe and who feel threatened by their illness are likely to be motivated to work in rehabilitation. However, severity and susceptibility is a double-edged sword and must be evaluated carefully. Motivation may be lowest for patients who feel that nothing can be done to improve their symptoms. For such patients, motivation is often enhanced by beginning a pulmonary rehabilitation program.

The third component, perceived benefits of and barriers to behavior change, is perhaps the most critical to evaluate. By definition, the perceived benefits of health behavior change must outweigh the costs or barriers before a patient is likely to undertake rehabilitation. Open and honest discussion with the patient at the outset of rehabilitation regarding the perceived benefits and costs of rehabilitation will be essential for determining the patient's level of motivation as well as the possible areas to address to increase motivation. Often motivation can be sparked in the reluctant patient if the most bothersome symptom is addressed during initial contact or if a special activity that the patient wants to regain is made to seem reachable. See figure 5.3 for a summary of the influence of the Health Belief Model on motivation.

Figure 5.3   Health Belief Model and Motivation

Cue to Action (e.g., doctor giving COPD diagnosis)
↑ motivation if presented with a hopeful message ("Your pulmonary tests are abnormal, but you still have a lot to work with.")
↓ motivation if told there is no cure ("There is no cure for emphysema.")

Perceived Severity or Susceptibility
↑ motivation if feeling slightly threatened ("If you continue to smoke, your lungs will get worse.")
↓ motivation if feeling "hopeless" ("I've smoked for 40 years, so why quit now that the damage is done?")

Perceived Benefits and Barriers
↑ motivation if benefits seem to outweigh barriers ("Your hard work in rehabilitation will pay off with increased independence and energy.")
↓ motivation if barriers appear overwhelming ("I have no transportation to get to pulmonary rehabilitation.")

Another factor in understanding patient motivation is self-efficacy, or the patient's perception of his or her ability to perform the behavior.[16] In the rehabilitation context, patients must believe that they can perform at least some of the exercises before they will be sufficiently motivated to engage in pulmonary rehabilitation.[17] This can be demonstrated by providing patients with an opportunity to observe or take part in a brief exercise session at the initial meeting. Practitioners can also provide the prospective patient with examples of successful patients with similar disease and circumstances. Through this, patients may have a better perspective of their own illness and not feel as isolated. Motivation can be enhanced when realistic, measurable, and personally important goals are discussed and agreed on.

Tobacco Use

Tobacco use is a critical health behavior to address during pulmonary rehabilitation. Although most patients have quit smoking by the time they enter a pulmonary rehabilitation program, some patients still remain unable to quit. Although controversy exists, accepting smokers into pulmonary rehabilitation programs is reasonable providing they are willing to actively engage in smoking cessation.[18,19] Because smoking patients are in the minority in the pulmonary rehabilitation setting, the likely peer pressure to quit smoking may help with motivation in this area. Open nonjudgmental discussions of smoking cessation among patients in pulmonary rehabilitation can be a positive experience both for the patients who have been successful in quitting and for the patients who continue to smoke. Patients with continuing tobacco use who are deemed appropriate candidates for pulmonary rehabilitation should have this behavior assessed frequently as an important outcome measure.

To assess motivation for smoking cessation and the stage of readiness to change, the Health Behavior Model components outlined previously should be considered. In addition, the Stages of Change Model,[20] which examines the structure of change that underlies modifying problem behaviors through both self-mediated and treatment-facilitated techniques, can be applied. This model integrates both motivational and behavioral aspects of change and recognizes that change occurs over time with specific mechanisms involved at each level. There is broad empirical evidence that this model is effective in smoking cessation initiatives.[21] The model's five stages of change are precontemplation (not thinking of quitting in the next 6 months), contemplation (considering quitting in the next 6 months but not in the next 30 days), preparation (considering quitting during the next 30 days), action (setting a quit date), and maintenance (purposeful cessation). Over time, patients may move forward and backward through these five stages of change. Knowing the patient's current stage of change will help the provider decide how best to intervene. For example, during the precontemplation stage (not thinking of quitting in the next 6 months), the appropriate provider strategies would be to incorporate the five R's:

Relevance—Tailor advice and discussion to each patient

Risks—Outline the risks of continued smoking

Rewards—Outline the benefits of quitting

Roadblocks—Identify barriers to quitting

Repetition—Reinforce the motivational message at each visit; do not tell them how bad smoking is in a judgemental manner

However, during the preparation stage (considering quitting during the next 30 days), the provider might help in the following ways:

- Praise the patient's readiness.
- Review previous quit attempts.
- Help set a quit date.
- Reinforce the need for support.
- Suggest medications and local smoking cessation programs.

All health care professionals should incorporate the five A's into each health care visit with smokers:

ASK about use at each visit.

ADVISE users to quit.

ASSESS readiness to quit.

ASSIST with their quit attempt.

ARRANGE follow-up care.

For smokers, bupropion hydrochloride, nicotine replacement therapy (NRT) in the form of gum, a transdermal patch, or a nasal spray may also be helpful. However, for optimum effectiveness and highest quit rates, NRT should be combined with a behavior modification program and social support.[22] NRT treatment options are listed in table 5.1.

Often smokers will indicate that they are motivated to quit because another person (physician, spouse, child) wants them to quit. Although support from external sources is important, the smoker must identify his or her own personal smoking cessation goals to help increase self-efficacy and sustain motivation.

Adherence to Medical Regimens

Adherence is a multifaceted, complex issue, and its assessment is not a simple task. Despite this challenge, a realistic assessment of adherence is essential to making accurate adjustments in the

Table 5.1 Treatment Options at a Glance

Product	Treatment period	Dosage	Pros	Cons
Nicotine patches	Preferably 8 weeks (at least 4)	21 mg or 15 mg for heavier smokers, 10 mg for lighter smokers; choose between 24- and 16-hr patches	• Very easy to use • Automatically gives the right dose • 24-hr patches can help with early morning cravings • Not addictive in the long term	• 24-hr patches may disturb sleep • Not orally gratifying • Small possibility of skin reaction
Nicotine gum	At least 4 weeks, then as needed	4 mg for heavy smokers, 2 mg for lighter smokers; 10-15 pieces a day	• Easy to regulate dose • Can prevent over-eating • Gives extra help at difficult moments	• Tricky with dentures • Need to use correctly
Nicotine spray	Up to 8 weeks, then reduce dose by 50% for 2 weeks	Dose once or twice an hour as required; don't use more than 64 sprays in 24 hours	• Gives fast relief to heavy smokers • Easy to adjust dose	• May cause nasal irritation at first • Dependence more likely • Doctor's help needed
Nicotine inhaler	Up to 8 weeks, then reduce dose by 50% for 2 weeks	6 to 12 cartridges per day	• Helps keep hands and mouth busy • Easy to regulate dose • Could help prevent overeating	• May not suffice for heavy smokers if used alone • May attract attention when used in public
Bupropion (Zyban)	7 to 12 weeks; start taking 8 to 14 days before quitting smoking	Day 1 to 3: 1 × 150 mg tablet each morning Day 4 on: 1 × 150 mg tablet A.M. and P.M.	• Good short-term research results • Easy to use • Noticeable reduction in urges to smoke	• Possible sleep disruption • May cause headaches and dry mouth

Adapted, by permission, from *STOP! Magazine*.

exercise, medication, or treatment regimen. Until recently, providers believed that if a course of action were recommended, the patient would judiciously follow it. Adherence was considered to be the total responsibility of the patient. Often, the patient's desire to please the physician overrode the importance of telling the truth. However, if the interaction occurs in a climate of shared responsibility, dignity, and respect, evaluation of adherence will be more accurate and objective.

The many factors influencing patient adherence to prescribed regimens include the following:[23,24]

- Beliefs and cultural norms
- Denial of a health problem
- Lack of understanding of the purpose of the regimen

- Complex medication regimen and administration route
- Forgetting
- Feeling better or feeling worse
- Undesirable side effects
- Concurrent illness or turmoil in the family
- Inability to access health care (e.g., problems with transportation, scheduling, referral process, insurance coverage)
- Perception of adverse provider–client relationship (dissatisfaction with the provider's competence, communication style, or personal qualities)
- Inability to deal with the cost of the medical regimen

- Extended disease course
- Unwillingness or inability to change comfortable habits or automatic behaviors
- No energy to invest in change

Adherence to rehabilitation programs among patients with a chronic illness is positively associated with the following characteristics:[25]

- Older age
- Higher socioeconomic status
- Better education
- Adaptive coping style
- Being married
- Stable lifestyle
- Abstinence from alcohol and smoking
- Decreased depression

Keeping these factors in mind when conducting a thorough and compassionate assessment of the potential for adherence to the medical regimen will give direction to the most successful plan and interventions.

Psychosocial Interventions

The psychosocial impact of coping with chronic respiratory disease can be devastating because the disease affects nearly all aspects of daily living. As the downward spiral begins, each aspect of coping with the disease presents a new challenge to overcome. The adequate management of any chronic illness encompasses a number of broad principles that address several universal problems. The chronic illness framework[26] outlined in figure 5.4 provides a comprehensive guide that speaks to the multiple problems of living daily with chronic lung disease. The patient and family will appreciate the all-inclusive approach to their care offered during pulmonary rehabilitation.

All patients with chronic respiratory disease are likely to benefit from some supportive counseling addressing one or more areas of concern (e.g., sexuality, anxiety, social support). Interventions may be provided in a one-on-one or group format, depending on the intensity of patient distress and the availability of therapeutic resources. Counseling and psychosocial support can be delivered by an experienced and designated member of the pulmonary rehabilitation team as a focused topic (e.g., a stress management module) or during the course of

---

Figure 5.4 Strauss' Framework of Chronic Illness Management

- Helping patients prevent and manage medical crises (e.g., providing education on infection and fluid overload)
- Helping patients control symptoms (e.g., teaching self-care strategies such as pursed-lip breathing, energy conservation, work simplification, and stress reduction)
- Managing medical regimen (e.g., setting mutually acceptable, realistic goals and modifing them as needed)
- Preventing social isolation (e.g., reinforcing strategies that increase confidence in social situations, such as pacing activities, panic control, and secretion clearance)
- Helping patients adjust to the trajectory of the disease (offering support groups, counseling, coping skills)
- Helping patients normalize their lifestyles (e.g., offering them a mechanism by which to vent their frustrations and express their concerns over time)
- Facilitating funding (e.g., considering the patient's ability to afford medications, suggesting less costly medications and treatments, and referring the patient to appropriate social services)
- Assisting with family adjustment to the chronic illness (e.g., validating the emotional turmoil of the spouse and close family, referring to psychological professionals for difficult family or marital issues)

---

other rehabilitative activities (e.g., during breathing retraining). As noted previously, patients experiencing significant emotional distress (e.g., depression) should be referred for further evaluation to an appropriate mental health practitioner, such as a clinical social worker, psychiatric nurse, psychologist, chaplain, or psychiatrist. In such patients, subsequent treatment efforts within pulmonary rehabilitation should be coordinated with the patient's primary care or mental health provider.

Building Support Systems

The psychosocial intervention perhaps most fundamental to pulmonary rehabilitation is developing an adequate support system.[27] Staff support, consisting of caring professionals displaying counseling skills, is key to successful programs. Such services often entail active listening and crisis management skills as well as patient advocacy and facilitation of resource acquisition.

Additional support may be derived from family members, friends, and other program participants. Generally speaking, patients with chronic respiratory disease who have positive social support have less depression and anxiety.[28] Studies have also shown that living with a partner is associated with an additional 12 months of life in patients with COPD.[29] Social support can be enhanced through educational presentations and patient involvement in support groups that encourage the sharing of personal rehabilitation experiences. The group environment is conducive to participant sharing of disease-related information and successful coping skills. It also provides an outlet for emotional release and elicitation of emotional support. Further opportunities for patient interaction can be developed in waiting areas and during social events. To enhance their sense of self-worth, some patients may also choose to serve as volunteers for the rehabilitation program or other community activities. It is important to note that some patients do not do well in a group setting; the pulmonary rehabilitation staff must respect each patient's sense of privacy.

Social support can also be fostered through the involvement of the patient's spouse or support person. Significant others should be encouraged to participate in support groups in which family dynamics and interpersonal skills can be observed, information can be shared, misperceptions can be clarified, and fears and concerns can be addressed. Practitioners should be sensitive to the caregiver or spouse because they are often receiving little support themselves.[30] Particularly important are discussions and skills development activities focusing on how family members can provide support to the patient without promoting dependency. Collaboration between the patient and support person is fostered when both parties can come to terms with the illness; commit to working together to manage the illness; be sensitive to cues signaling the needs, desires, and feelings of the other; compromise; and seek out choices and resources for managing their lives.[31] For the patient having significant interpersonal or family conflict, referral to a clinical social worker, psychologist, or other counselor for family or relationship counseling is recommended.

Managing Stress

Stress management training should include an easily understood, practical model for describing the effects of stress on the mind and body. Patients should be trained to recognize their own early warning signs and symptoms of stress (e.g., anxiety, dyspnea, muscle tension) and be capable

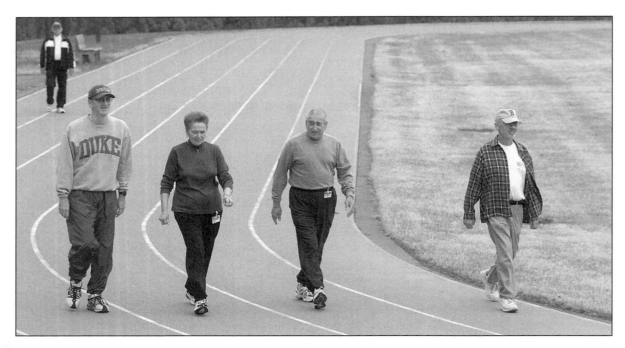

Pulmonary rehabilitation patients need good social support. Friends, spouses, children, grandchildren, and the rehabilitation staff all provide needed support.

of performing a variety of stress management techniques. Relaxation training for the mind and body can be accomplished through progressive muscle relaxation, imagery, autogenics, and yoga. To reinforce the training, relaxation tapes may be provided for home use. Relaxation practice may be supplemented through biofeedback. It is imperative that relaxation training be integrated into the patient's daily routine with specific application to dyspnea and panic control.

Because patients with chronic pulmonary disease often experience medical or other life crises, crisis management skills are useful. Appropriate interventions may include the following:

- Conveying empathy through active listening
- Teaching calming exercises (e.g., breathing retraining techniques)
- Offering anticipatory guidance regarding upcoming stressors
- Assisting the patient with problem solving
- Identifying resources and support systems[32]

These interventions should be used in a manner that would not encourage excessive patient dependency. In an effort to be as helpful as possible, pul-monary rehabilitation staff might inadvertently promote patient dependence rather than independence.

Treating Significant Emotional Distress

Anxiety and depression are common in patients with advanced chronic respiratory disease. In a group of 243 lung transplant candidates, five different personality styles emerged on the Minnesota Multiphasic Personality Inventory (MMPI). The majority of patients evidenced mild somatic and mood disturbances. Almost one fourth exhibited marked anxiety and mood disturbances, and a small cluster evidenced features consistent with an antisocial personality style.[33] Unfortunately, these comorbid conditions are frequently under-recognized and undertreated.[34,35] Furthermore, even when appropriate treatment is recommended, many patients refuse antianxiety or antidepressant medication because of fear of side effects, embarrassment, denial of the illness, worries about addiction, cost concerns, or a frustration with taking too many drugs.[36] Subthreshold depression, described as clinically relevant depression that does not fit

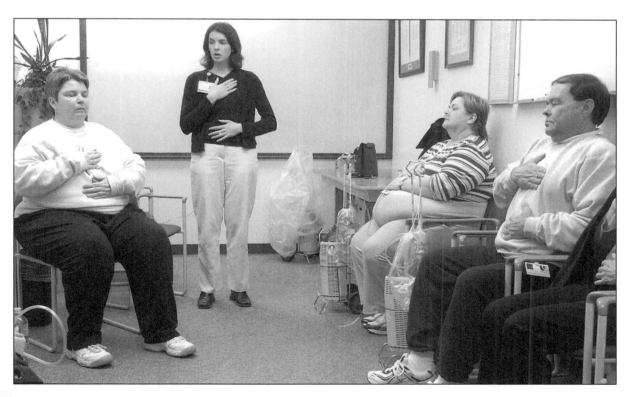

Learning relaxation techniques helps a patient manage stress, and managing stress is key to a successful pulmonary rehabilitation program.

operational criteria, is seen in 25% of elderly patients with COPD.[37] Patients who have significant impairment as a result of depression, anxiety, anger, or hostility should be referred to a mental health professional experienced in working with patients who have chronic illness.

Addressing Issues of Sexuality

Sexual functioning is affected by chronic illness in a variety of ways. The patient–spouse relationship, degree of affection, communication, and level of satisfaction with his or her partner is most frequently problematic. In one report more than 67% of COPD patients studied showed some type of sexual problem.[38] This sensitive topic of sexuality needs to be addressed because it is often a topic of utmost importance for quality of life. Being sexually active has been shown to actually improve physiologic functioning in patients with noninvasive mechanical ventilation.[39] If sexuality is approached in a straightforward and factual way, it will not be embarrassing to the clinician or the patient. Although general information may be provided during patient education in a small-group format, specific questions and concerns are generally best addressed in a one-on-one or couples format. An outline of topics that may be appropriate to discuss with patients is presented in figure 5.5. The pulmonary rehabilitation specialist may be effective in facilitating the discussion and resolution of sexual issues with many patients. Patients or their partners experiencing significant emotional distress, however, or long-term difficulties with intimacy or sexual dysfunction should be referred to an appropriate mental health provider.

Strategies to Improve Adherence to the Exercise Prescription

The following strategies to improve adherence have been used with varying degrees of success by many practitioners. Choose the behavioral interventions that might work best for each patient and with which you feel most comfortable. The majority of the strategies will result in improved adherence, but there is no one perfect strategy. You may want to try several interventions and use the one that works the best and costs the least.

- Using exercise logs outlining intensity, duration, and frequency of home exercise
- Reviewing exercise progress weekly in person (one on one), by phone, or by e-mail

---

Figure 5.5 Issues to Address in Sexual Counseling With Lung Patients

Biological Issues
- Variations of sexual performance problems
- Effects of the aging process
- Sexual effects of organic factors related to the illness
- Is sexual activity safe?
- Effects of medications
- Evaluation and treatment options

Behavioral Factors
- Setting the appropriate sexual context
- Specific sexual technique

Emotional Factors
- Importance of relaxation and comfort
- Sexual effects of antierotic emotions

Cognitive Factors
- Anxiety-provoking beliefs
- Myths versus realities

Personality Factors
- Need for education, permission, or therapy

Relationship Factors
- Issues that relate to overall intimacy
- Sex versus sexuality in context

Sensory Factors
- Sensate focus as an antidote to anxiety
- Advisability of self-stimulation

Reprinted, by permission, from W.M. Sotile, 1996, *Psychosocial interventions for cardiopulmonary patients: A guide for health professionals* (Champaign, IL: Human Kinetics), 209.

- Emphasizing the symptom relief achieved as endurance gains are made
- Creating a mutually determined and signed written agreement, including projected dates of accomplishment
- Reestablishing goals after initial goals are met
- Setting up systems of reminders (calls from friends, calendars, refrigerator magnet notes)
- Identifying an exercise component that will best help the patient to meet a coveted personal goal and emphasize work in that area

- Fitting the plan to the patient's daily routine and simplifying it as much as possible
- Encouraging the patient to return to the program (repeating it if necessary) as soon as possible after an exacerbation

Promoting Long-Term Adherence to Lifestyle Changes

Pulmonary rehabilitation is not simply a brief program with a beginning and an end, but a commitment to a lifestyle change. Cognitive and behavioral interventions can be useful in helping patients to adhere to the recommended lifestyle modifications (e.g., diet, exercise, refraining from substance abuse).[40] Adherence to exercise is particularly important because it has been shown to enhance psychological adjustment, reduce anxiety, and improve cognitive performance and endurance in patients with COPD.[41-45]

Overall, studies of short-term pulmonary rehabilitation programs in patients with chronic respiratory disease have consistently shown positive outcomes that last for at least one year.[19] Studies of specific longer-term interventions have shown promising but mixed results. Many questions remain unanswered as to the optimal strategies for maximizing longer-term outcomes.

A major challenge to the pulmonary rehabilitation community is to develop successful strategies for extending positive outcomes beyond the formal program. A major barrier to administering quality long-term maintenance programs is the current lack of reimbursement for this activity. If long-term improvement is to be maintained, adherence to exercise must be encouraged through ongoing reinforcement. Practical models for long-term training that provide intermittent reinforcement,[43] gradual weaning of sessions, booster sessions,[46] repeat programs[47], distractive auditory stimuli,[48] longer programs,[49] and intensive home training[50] have shown promise. The addition of a support group and telephone calls three months after the completion of a program did not make a significant difference in health status or walking distance in one comparative study.[51] Exacerbations of COPD appear to be important factors negatively affecting long-term adherence to rehabilitation recommendations. After an exacerbation and a decrease in functional status, referral back to formal rehabilitation may be appropriate.

Emphasis should be placed on relapse prevention strategies that have been shown to facilitate long-term behavior change.[52] Because adherence is

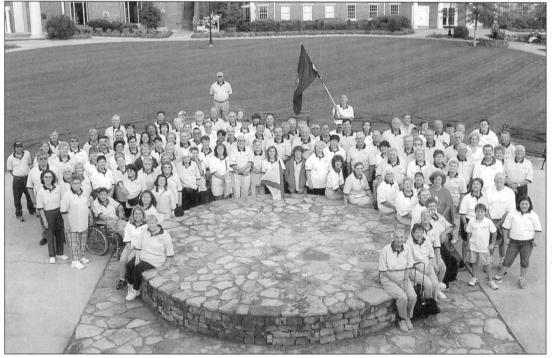

Photo courtesy of AACVPR.

The first AACVPR Heart/Lung Games, held in 2003, was an opportunity for fellowship and friendly athletic competition. Such competitions are also a way to encourage life-long adherence to a rehabilitation program.

influenced by multidimensional and complex factors, treatment strategies must be multifocused. No single strategy can work for everyone. Therapeutic strategies that should be integrated into every aspect of the rehabilitation program are as follows:

- Asking patients early in each visit what concerns they have about their lung problem and what they want to address during the visit.

- Enhancing patients' understanding and "ownership" of each component of the treatment regimen. Practitioners can discuss ways in which newly acquired behaviors might fit into patients' daily schedules.

- Developing patients' ability to identify situations in which they are likely to be at high risk of relapse (e.g., failing to maintain the exercise regimen, reverting back to the anxiety/dyspnea attack cycle, misusing medications, smoking) and brainstorming solutions with them.

- Promoting patients' ability to solve problems independently as they arise during daily living; providing appropriate praise for attempts and accomplishments (improves self-esteem); and reinforcing positive experiences.

- Encouraging involvement by the patient and family in structured social support activities (e.g., church, clubs, exercise programs, volunteer activities).

- Reassessing the patient's commitment to adherence at discharge, prior to generating the recommended home exercise and treatment plan.

Conclusion

A strong, trusting bond must be established with patients early in pulmonary rehabilitation to ensure successful outcomes. Assessment for psychosocial issues should be routinely performed at the outset of pulmonary rehabilitation. Intervention, when necessary, should be integrated into the comprehensive treatment plan. Although the psychosocial needs of individual patients vary widely, in general, a minimum of four hours would be appropriate for most patients. The use of a chronic illness framework will help to organize the approach to the multidimensional issues involved. Psychosocial interventions, offered in either individual or group formats, can be effective in reducing distress and facilitating adaptive coping. Breathing retraining, relaxation training, and stress management training can be beneficial in reducing the anxiety/dyspnea cycle and should be an integral part of the overall treatment plan. Patients experiencing substantial impairments in psychological functioning should be referred to a mental health provider for further evaluation and treatment. Reassessment of psychological status and refinement of interventions is an essential component of discharge planning. Developing a plan for the maintenance of activities that promote and reinforce the strategies learned will be useful in the long-term maintenance of physiologic and psychosocial gains.[53]

chapter 6

Outcome Assessment

Pulmonary rehabilitation often results in a substantial decrease in dyspnea and fatigue, an increase in exercise performance, and an improvement in functional status and health status. The purpose of outcome assessment in pulmonary rehabilitation is to measure these and other changes objectively. As the environment of health care evolves toward reducing cost, more efficiently managing care, deleting duplication of services, and enhancing the quality of life, outcome assessment has become an increasingly important component of pulmonary rehabilitation.

Because pulmonary rehabilitation involves the interaction of the patient with an interdisciplinary team of professionals, outcome assessment can have differing goals and perspectives. The goals of the patient and his or her perceived success of the intervention in achieving these goals may differ from those of the pulmonary rehabilitation staff, the insurance providers, and even society. A listing of the reasons for assessing outcomes in pulmonary rehabilitation is given in figure 6.1.

Timing of Patient-Centered Outcome Measurement

Outcome measurement in pulmonary rehabilitation requires the evaluation of changes in improvement variables resulting from this rehabilitation. At a minimum, pre- and postrehabilitation changes should be assessed. However, assessment of long-term changes may also be desirable.

Figure 6.1 Reasons for Outcome Assessment in Pulmonary Rehabilitation

- Outcome assessment documents the effectiveness of the intervention for the individual patient and the patient group as a whole.
- The patient-to-patient variability in improvement following pulmonary rehabilitation in all outcome areas is substantial, making individual documentation of outcomes necessary.
- Direct, positive feedback on the achievement of specific goals during rehabilitation may serve to increase the morale and motivation of both the patient and the pulmonary rehabilitation staff.
- The evaluation of multiple outcomes provides valuable feedback to rehabilitation staff on the effectiveness of the various components of the program. This may be used for continuous quality improvement.
- Traditional physiologic indices of severity such as the FEV_1 do not change appreciably with pulmonary rehabilitation, and they cannot serve as surrogate markers for improvement in areas of importance to the patient, such as relief of dyspnea or improvement in health status.
- The objective assessment of health care use outcomes provides information on the cost effectiveness of pulmonary rehabilitation; this is of obvious importance to third-party payers and facility administration.
- Assessment of pre- to postrehabilitation outcomes of importance to the patient can provide useful information on the success of the individual pulmonary rehabilitation program.
- Objective data on the progress of the individual patient provide important feedback information to the referring physician.

Pre- to Postrehabilitation Assessment of Outcomes

Patient-centered outcomes must be measured objectively to evaluate the progress of the patient and the effectiveness of the pulmonary rehabilitation program. This is usually accomplished by measuring specific outcomes immediately before pulmonary rehabilitation starts and then shortly after the end of the program (pre- and postrehabilitation assessment). The same instrument should be used "pre" and "post" to document change.

Long-Term Assessment of Outcomes

Some of the benefits achieved during the rehabilitation process wane over time following the end of the formal pulmonary rehabilitation process. Because of this, many programs now incorporate a maintenance plan, individualized to the patient, following pulmonary rehabilitation. This plan may include reinforcement in ongoing exercise, self-care skills, education, and support. This has the added benefit of encouraging patients to stay connected to the professional rehabilitation staff. Because of the potential drop-off in gains with time and the fact that a prominent goal of pulmonary rehabilitation is to maintain the benefits in the long term, longitudinal assessment of outcomes should be considered. A reasonable timing for these might be at six-month intervals for a year or two. This longitudinal assessment has the potential benefit of identifying those patients with substantial decreases in outcome areas, who would be candidates for reenrollment in formal

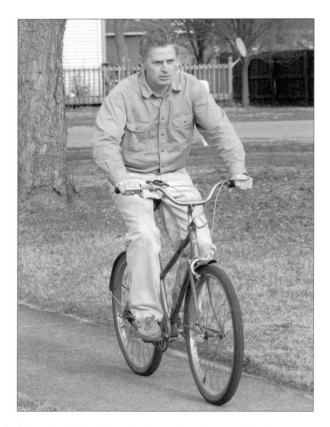

For rehabilitation to be effective, patients must continue to follow the program, even after formal rehabilitation is over. Finding exercises that patients can do on their own is vital to successful long-term program adherence.

pulmonary rehabilitation. Long-term assessment can be in several outcome areas such as health-related quality of life, dyspnea, and exercise performance.

Domains for Outcome Assessment

The Outcomes Committee of the AACVPR has identified four domains of outcome assessment: health, clinical, behavioral, and service, as outlined in table 6.1.

Outcome assessment in specific, measurable areas is considered an essential component of comprehensive pulmonary rehabilitation (ATS statement).[1] Accordingly, the AACVPR Guidelines Committee recommends as a minimum the assessment of outcomes in all domains, both pre- and postpulmonary rehabilitation. The longer-term assessment of outcomes, at 6 and 12 months, although not mandatory, is encouraged. The type of outcome assessment usually depends on the goals and requirements (e.g., individual clinical patient assessments, program continuous quality improvement, clinical research), staffing, and resources of the individual program.

Health Domain

The health domain includes the outcome areas of morbidity, mortality, and health-related quality of life (health status). For the individual clinically oriented pulmonary rehabilitation program, health-related quality of life is a relevant outcome that is easily measured and often shows impressive change with treatment. Mortality and morbidity (which includes health care use, loss of workdays, and missed rehabilitation visits), although of obvious importance, are difficult for the individual program to measure and analyze.

Health-Related Quality of Life

A prominent goal of pulmonary rehabilitation is to improve health-related quality of life, or health status, according to the American Thoracic Society (ATS).[1] Therefore, measurement of outcome in this essential area is of importance to the pulmonary rehabilitation program. Quality of life can be defined as "the gap between that which is desired in life and that which is achieved."[1,2,3] It is affected by factors other than health or disease, such as job and financial security, housing, family and relationships, and spirituality. Health-related quality of life is narrower in scope, focusing on just those areas of quality of life affected by health. Its measurement in pulmonary rehabilitation quantifies the impact of the respiratory disease, its comorbidity, and treatment side effects on the patient's daily life activities and sense of well-being. Health-related quality of life questionnaires for patients with respiratory disease usually have multiple dimensions or domains, often assessing functional status, symptoms (especially dyspnea and fatigue), the feeling of mastery over the disease, the impact of the disease on the person, and overall satisfaction or dissatisfaction with life.

Questionnaires that measure health-related quality of life can be generic or respiratory specific. The former assess overall health in any disease, or even in healthy individuals, and the latter assess health only in individuals with a specific respiratory disease such as chronic obstructive pulmonary disease (COPD). Generic instruments provide information on factors other than respiratory disease (such as pain) that might influence health. The narrower focus in disease-specific instruments usually makes them very helpful tools in assessing change with therapy—a useful feature for assessing outcome in pulmonary rehabilitation.

The health-related quality of life questionnaire for pulmonary rehabilitation should be valid (measure what it says it measures), reliable (be

Table 6.1 Outcome Assessment Domains*

Outcome domain	Performance indicators
Health	Health-related quality of life (health status), survival
Clinical	Exertional dyspnea, dyspnea with daily activities, fatigue, exercise performance, depression or anxiety
Behavioral	Smoking cessation, breathing retraining, coping strategies, bronchial hygiene, medication adherence, supplemental oxygen use, pacing technique, energy conservation, sexual function, adherence to diet
Service	Patient satisfaction

* Please refer to the pulmonary rehabilitation outcome matrix in the members only section of the AACVPR Web site (www.aacvpr.org) for a complete listing of indicators.

reproducible over multiple measurements), and have good evaluative properties (be able to detect change with therapy). In addition, it should be short, easy for the patient to read and understand, and easy for the staff to administer. Ideally it should be self-administered. Patients, not staff members or spouses, should complete health-related questionnaires.

For patients with COPD undergoing pulmonary rehabilitation, the interviewer-administered Chronic Respiratory Disease Questionnaire (CRQ, or CRDQ)[4] and its newer, self-administered version[5] have many of the previously described important features and should be useful to many pulmonary rehabilitation programs. The 20-item CRQ has four domains: dyspnea (five items), fatigue (four items), emotion (seven items), and mastery—the feeling of control over the disease (four items). In addition, a total score can be calculated. Although the questions pertaining to fatigue, emotion, and mastery are standardized, the five dyspnea items are unique to the patient. For these, the patient identifies five activities that were frequently performed and caused dyspnea in the past 2 weeks. A list of activities is provided for suggestions, or the patient can choose unique activities. Each of the five dyspnea-producing activities and the 15 standardized items in the other domains are scored using a seven-point scale, with higher scores indicating higher levels of health. A 0.5-unit-per-question change resulting from therapy is considered a clinically meaningful change. The self-administered version is easier to administer, maintaining the desirable features of the instrument.

Other examples of validated respiratory quality of life questionnaires that might be useful for pulmonary rehabilitation are the St. George's Respiratory Questionnaire (SGRQ) and the Ferrans & Powers QOL—Pulmonary Version. The AACVPR Outcomes Resource Guide in the members only section of the Web site (www.aacvpr.org) is currently under revision but will have more detailed descriptions of these and other instruments.

COPD-specific instruments such as the CRQ or SGRQ have not been validated for the entire spectrum of respiratory diseases (such as interstitial lung disease or primary pulmonary hypertension) seen in pulmonary rehabilitation. For these patients, a generic tool such as the Medical Outcomes Study Short-Form 36 would be appropriate. Generic instruments also would be useful to capture some of the disturbance in health status caused by comorbid conditions. Because of these considerations, some programs may wish to consider using a generic instrument to complement a respiratory-specific instrument.

Morbidity and Mortality

Morbidity and mortality, although of paramount importance, do not lend themselves to easy evaluation by the individual pulmonary rehabilitation program. Variables such as survival or health care resource use are often best suited for multicenter studies, but can be used in individual programs if so desired.

Clinical Domain

The clinical domain predominantly reflects the physical and psychological changes resulting from pulmonary rehabilitation but is also influenced by patient behaviors and lifestyle changes. Measurable outcome areas in this domain include the symptoms of dyspnea and fatigue, exercise performance, and the psychological variables of anxiety and depression.

Dyspnea

Dyspnea is usually the overriding symptom in COPD patients referred to pulmonary rehabilitation and is the most influential factor affecting health-related quality of life. Although dyspnea is subjective and complex, it nonetheless must be measured objectively. In pulmonary rehabilitation outcome assessment, two general forms of dyspnea assessment can be performed: (1) rating exertional breathlessness during a specific task, such as during exercise testing or a timed distance walk, and (2) rating the overall level of breathlessness during daily activities. Figure 6.2 lists commonly used dyspnea scales.

For rating exertional dyspnea, the 10-point Borg scale used during a specified task (such as a 6-

---

Figure 6.2 Examples of Dyspnea Measurements in Pulmonary Rehabilitation

Exertional Dyspnea
Borg Scale[7]
VAS (Visual Analog Scale)[8]
Overall Breathlessness With Activities
BDI/TDI (Baseline Dyspnea Index/Transitional Dyspnea Index)[9,10]
UCSD Shortness of Breath Questionnaire[11]
Modified Medical Research Council (MRC) Questionnaire[12,13]
Dyspnea domain of the CRQ
Dyspnea components of the Pulmonary Functional Status Scale (PFSS)[14] and Modified Pulmonary Functional Status and Dyspnea Questionnaire (PFSDQ-M)[15,16]

minute timed distance walk) is an easy-to-perform, accepted, and reliable assessment. For rating overall dyspnea with daily activities, the patient-specific dyspnea domain of the CRQ has been extensively used in pulmonary rehabilitation and has proven very sensitive in detecting change with pulmonary rehabilitation. Its use also provides assessment in other domains comprising health-related quality of life. Alternative tools for this measurement might be the University of California at San Diego (UCSD) Shortness of Breath Questionnaire or the Baseline and Transitional Dyspnea Indexes (BDI and TDI). Both the UCSD Shortness of Breath Questionnaire and the BDI/TDI are easy to administer and have been able to detect improvement in this symptom following pulmonary rehabilitation.

Exercise Performance

Tests of exercise performance can vary from simple field tests of exercise performance, such as the 6-minute walk test, to complex cardiopulmonary exercise tests with measurement of gas exchange.

Field Tests of Exercise Performance

Exercise training is an essential component of pulmonary rehabilitation, and outcome assessment of exercise performance is mandatory. The type of exercise evaluation in pulmonary rehabilitation can range from simple to complex, depending on the program, its staffing, and resource capabilities. However, any pulmonary rehabilitation program should have at minimum the resources and staffing to perform a field test of exercise performance, such

as the 6-minute walk test, before and at the end of the program.

The popularity of the 6-minute walk test in outcome assessment for pulmonary rehabilitation probably results from several factors: (1) It is easy to administer and requires no special equipment; (2) the type, duration, and intensity of the exercise are relevant to many activities of daily living; (3) the walk test has documented improvement following pulmonary rehabilitation; and (4) a clinically meaningful change in the 6-minute walk distance (~52 meters) has been established.

The 6-minute walk test is potentially biased by practice attempts and encouragement by the rehabilitation personnel. Because of this, strict standardization is highly recommended. To help with standardization, a copy of the American Thoracic Society Statement Guidelines for the Six-Minute Walk Test is included in appendix C. These guidelines provide valuable instructions that should help standardize this outcome measure. The AACVPR Guidelines Committee endorses these ATS guidelines for the 6-minute walk, but recommends that measurement of oxygen saturation during the testing not be optional but mandatory. Additionally, safety reasons may require that a staff member walk behind the patient during the testing.

The shuttle walk test is another field test of exercise ability.[17] This incremental walk test requires the patient to traverse a 10-meter distance, set by marker cones, at gradually increasing speeds. Instructions are given to walk at a steady pace with a goal of reaching the opposite marker cone at the next beeping signal from the cassette player.

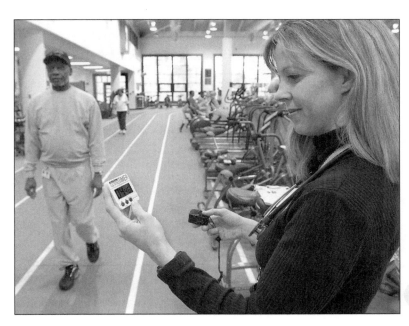

The 6-minute walk test is an excellent way to assess exercise outcomes.

The initial speed required is 0.5 meters/second, but is increased after every minute of walking by shortening the time between beeping signals. The test end point is determined when the patient becomes too breathless to keep up with the pace or is unable to complete the shuttle in the time allowed. The total distance (number of completed shuttles multiplied by 10 meters) is calculated. The newer endurance shuttle walk test requires walking the same course at a preset submaximal walking speed.[18] The shuttle walk tests require less space than the 6-minute walk test, and the potential confounding effects of pacing differences are essentially eliminated. However, unlike the 6-minute walk test, some special equipment is needed.

Laboratory Tests of Exercise Performance

There are two forms of exercise testing in the laboratory setting: incremental up to a maximum and submaximal steady state exercise, usually at a high fraction of maximum rate. Complexity increases with breath-by-breath analysis of ventilation and expiratory gases, arterial blood gas analysis, and measurements of spirometry and lung volumes.

Incremental cardiopulmonary exercise testing on a stationary cycle or treadmill, combined with the measurement of exhaled gases and tidal volume, provides considerable physiologic data and is useful in demonstrating the physiologic changes resulting from exercise training. Additional, important advantages of this assessment tool are that it allows the rehabilitation staff to evaluate maximal exercise performance, develop an exercise prescription, screen for underlying cardiac disease and orthopedic problems, and determine exercise hypoxemia. Measurements of heart rate, respiratory rate, oxygen saturation, blood pressure, level of dyspnea, and electrocardiographic tracings are routinely monitored. Analysis of expired gases allows for the determination or calculation of variables, such as oxygen consumption, carbon dioxide production, minute ventilation, and anaerobic threshold. This gives information on cardiovascular, ventilatory, and gas exchange limitations to maximal exercise performance and can help in determining if a physiologic training response occurred following exercise training.

Endurance testing can be done using a stationary cycle, ergometer, or treadmill at a high fraction of work rate determined by incremental testing. Changes in endurance time at equivalent work rates are often substantial following pulmonary rehabilitation exercise training. Like incremental testing, endurance testing allows practitioners to

---

> **Figure 6.3** Tests of Exercise Performance
>
> **Field Tests**
> Timed walk distance test (6-minute walk test)
> Shuttle walk test (incremental and endurance)
> **Laboratory Tests**
> Incremental cardiopulmonary exercise test
> Submaximal endurance test

analyze clinical and physiologic data concurrently. Incremental and submaximal endurance testing are described in chapter 4. Figure 6.3 summarizes tests of exercise performance.

Psychological Status

Patients with chronic respiratory disease often have significant associated anxiety and depression. Screening for these psychological issues is important in the initial pulmonary rehabilitation evaluation, and the measurement of changes in the psychological domain is an appropriate outcome assessment. The Guidelines Committee recommends routine screening for depression and anxiety by clinical evaluation or questionnaire, and the measurement of outcome in this area for those with identified problems. The Beck Depression Inventory, the CES-D, and the Hospital Anxiety and Depression (HAD) questionnaire are useful instruments in this area of assessment and outcome.

Cognitive Function

Patients with chronic respiratory disease can demonstrate cognitive impairment involving memory, attention and concentration, and problem-solving abilities during daily activities. Such impairment may interfere with all aspects of the rehabilitation process. Cognitive impairment can affect the ability to take medications correctly, learn breathing exercises, follow exercise instruction in the rehabilitation facility and at home, and benefit from the educational sessions. Evaluation of cognitive dysfunction should be considered as a screening test and an outcome tool. Cognitive impairment is discussed in chapter 5.

Functional Performance

Functional performance, which refers to activities of daily living (ADLs), is often considerably reduced in patients with chronic respiratory disease. Basic ADLs include feeding, dressing, personal hygiene, bowel function, and physical mobility. Instrumental ADLs include more physically demanding work, including shopping, home chores, and housework. Patients with chronic respiratory disease often adapt to the dyspnea and fatigue associated with these activities by working at a slower pace or modifying the environment. One of the goals of pulmonary rehabilitation is to improve functional performance. This is accomplished through reducing dyspnea and improving exercise endurance, stamina, and pacing in ADLs. Outcome assessment for functional performance can be measured by questionnaire. Examples of respiratory-specific functional performance instruments include the PFSS[14] and the PFSDQ. [15,16]

Behavioral Domain

Observable changes in the behavioral domain are sometimes the most significant for the patient, but difficult to measure. To fairly judge the patient's progress in this domain, pre to post measurements are essential for documenting changes over the duration of the pulmonary rehabilitation program. Potential outcome areas in the behavioral domain are adherence to an exercise regimen, use of supplemental oxygen, progression with smoking cessation, and compliance with diet and medication instructions. In addition, other demonstrable changes such as the application of coping mechanisms, relaxation, stress management, breathing retraining, and pacing techniques can be measured. Potential outcome areas in the behavioral domain are listed in figure 6.4. Unfor-

---

Figure 6.4 Potential Outcome Areas in the Behavioral Domain

Knowledge of educational objectives (determined by testing)
Success with smoking cessation efforts
Adherence to diet instructions
Adherence to medications
Adherence to the exercise prescription
Adherence to postrehabilitation exercise directions
Adherence to breathing retraining
Supplemental oxygen use
Success with coping mechanisms
Success with energy conservation techniques
Success with relaxation and stress management techniques
Success with pacing techniques

---

tunately, very few formalized, validated tools are available to assess specific behavioral domain outcomes in pulmonary rehabilitation. Therefore, unlike the situation in the health and clinical domains, staff may have to design or adapt a tool that is relevant to its particular goals and patient population.

Service Domain

Pulmonary rehabilitation is a customer service program, and a major component of the job of the rehabilitation staff is to deliver excellent customer services to patients and their families as an

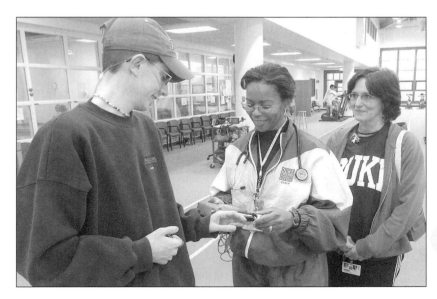

Perhaps the most important part of a rehabilitation program is the staff. A friendly, caring staff is vital to a good rehabilitation program.

extension of the physician's management. Evaluation of this service is best determined using a satisfaction survey at the end of pulmonary rehabilitation.

Conclusion

Along with assessment, education, exercise training, psychosocial support, and long-term maintenance and follow-up, outcome assessment is an integral component of the pulmonary rehabilitation program. This process should not be intimidating, burdensome, or excessively time consuming. For clinically oriented programs with limited resources and staff, a reasonable approach would be to select one assessment from each of the four domains. The instruments or tests chosen should depend on the experience and preferences of the individual program. Following is an example of an outcome assessment strategy:

- Measurement of health-related quality of life and dyspnea (health domain). The self-report version of the Chronic Respiratory Disease Questionnaire (CRQ-SR) measures both. (20 minutes of staff time)

- Measurement of exercise performance (clinical domain). The 6-minute walk test is easiest to administer. Measurement of exertional dyspnea can also be accomplished at this time using a Borg scale. (30 minutes of staff time)

- Clinical assessment and documentation in one of the areas of the behavioral domain or the administration of a knowledge questionnaire (behavioral domain). (30 minutes of staff time)

- Administration of a brief satisfaction survey (service domain). (5 minutes of staff time)

These basic outcome measurements can provide valuable feedback to the program staff, patient, referring physician, and administrators regarding individual patients' responses and the overall success of the program. This assessment can be accomplished in less than 1 1/2 hours' time at the beginning and completion of the program. Other outcome areas could be assessed depending on the expertise, goals, and resources of the program.

chapter 7

Disease-Specific Approaches in Pulmonary Rehabilitation

Chronic obstructive pulmonary disease (COPD) is the most common condition for which people are referred for pulmonary rehabilitation. Indeed, the vast majority of investigation demonstrating the clinical benefits and scientific rationale for pulmonary rehabilitation has been undertaken in this patient population. Among patients with COPD, significant and striking improvements in exercise tolerance, health-related quality of life, and dyspnea occur following pulmonary rehabilitation despite the presence of underlying irreversible structural lung disease. The severity of impairment in lung function is only one of several key factors that limit the functional capacity and exercise tolerance of these people. Several additional factors associated with chronic respiratory disease such as skeletal muscle dysfunction, nutritional depletion, obesity, cardiovascular limitation, chest wall abnormalities (including kyphoscoliosis, respiratory muscle dysfunction, and thoracic compression fractures as a result of osteoporosis), psychologic disturbances such as anxiety and depression, electrolyte disturbances, and anemia also contribute commonly to the functional limitation.

Skeletal muscle dysfunction is a particularly important cause of leg fatigue and discomfort, limiting exercise as well as reducing strength and exercise endurance.[1] Skeletal muscle dysfunction is also associated with reduced health-related quality of life and increased use of health care resources, and may be a risk factor for increased mortality.[1-3] Deconditioning, aging, systemic inflammation, corticosteroid use, and nutritional impairment are common causes of this skeletal muscle dysfunction in people with COPD.[1] Importantly, improvements in skeletal muscle function and management of the other comorbidities noted are the principal mechanisms by which patients with COPD improve following pulmonary rehabilitation (see chapter 1).

The associated morbidities mentioned previously are by no means unique to COPD, and in fact are common manifestations of several forms of chronic respiratory disease. The scientific rationale for administering pulmonary rehabilitation to people with many other diagnoses (although they are less studied to date) exists just as strongly as it does for patients with COPD. People with asthma, cystic fibrosis, chronic interstitial lung disease, obesity-related respiratory disease, neuromuscular and/or chest wall disorders, and pulmonary hypertension, as well as people with chronic respiratory disease in preparation for thoracic or upper abdominal surgery who lack clear contraindications to exercise can all benefit from pulmonary rehabilitation[4-9] (see figure 7.1). Although patients with non-COPD diagnoses have the potential to benefit from participation in a pulmonary rehabilitation program, they also pose new challenges for the rehabilitation professional. Although the general components of comprehensive pulmonary rehabilitation (i.e., assessment, patient education, exercise, psychosocial intervention, and follow-up) are the same for these patients as for the COPD population, modification of the way these components are used is essential to ensure patient safety and meet individual patient needs. In this chapter we will review the mechanisms of exercise intolerance and functional impairment for people with respiratory disease other than COPD and discuss the key issues specific to these diseases that must be considered and addressed during pulmonary rehabilitation.

Asthma

Asthma is a chronic inflammatory disorder of the airways characterized by episodic bronchoconstriction, airways hyperresponsiveness, and intermittent exacerbations of airflow obstruction. It differs from COPD in two important respects that affect the goals and implementation of pulmonary rehabilitation. First, in asthma, the airflow obstruction is completely reversible, and baseline pulmonary function is normal when the disease is well controlled in the majority of people. Therefore, maintenance of normal pulmonary function through proper self- and medical management, rather than control of symptoms, is a crucial goal. Second, exercise is a major stimulus leading to bronchoconstriction for many asthmatics,[10,11] and efforts to prevent or manage exercise-induced bronchoconstriction must therefore be incorporated into the rehabilitation program.

Dyspnea, cough, and wheezing are common symptoms of asthma. Asthma is a common cause of absenteeism from work and school, psychological distress and perceived low self-efficacy,[12] increased health care use, and impaired quality of life.[13,14] People with well-controlled asthma without permanent airflow obstruction can have normal cardiopulmonary responses to exercise.[11] However, patients vary in disease severity (baseline lung function, frequency and severity of exacerbations) and triggers for exacerbation. Moreover, individual patients also have variable degrees of airflow obstruction or exercise-induced bronchospasm over time that can affect exercise tolerance. People with active airflow obstruction may experience ventilatory limitation to exercise and may develop hyperinflation with faster respiratory rates that can lead to mechanical disadvantage of the respiratory

---

Figure 7.1   Conditions Other Than COPD for Which Pulmonary Rehabilitation May Be Helpful

Obstructive Lung Disease
Asthma
Cystic fibrosis
Bronchiectasis

Nonobstructive Respiratory Disease
Interstitial lung disease (including survivors of adult respiratory distress syndrome)
Obesity-related respiratory impairment
Pulmonary vascular disease and pulmonary hypertension
Neuromuscular and neurologic conditions (e.g., poststroke)
Restrictive chest wall disease

Other Conditions
Before and after lung volume reduction surgery
Before and after lung transplantation
Lung cancer and thoracic or abdominal surgery
Ventilator dependency
Coexisting respiratory and cardiac disease
Pediatric patients with respiratory disease

muscles. Anxiety, fear of exercise, deconditioning, obesity, and steroid-induced myopathy commonly contribute to the dyspnea and exercise intolerance experienced by asthmatics, particularly those with more severe disease. In general, people with asthma tend to be less physically fit than those who are unaffected.[12,15,16] Importantly, resting lung function is a poor predictor of exercise ventilation.[11] Therefore, cardiopulmonary exercise testing is particularly helpful in determining the causes of exercise intolerance and formulating the exercise prescription for individual asthmatic patients.

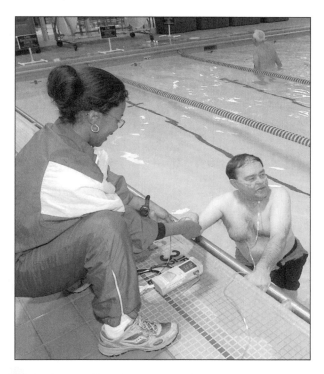

Individuals with asthma need to keep healthy lung functions through exercise. Exercises such as swimming or water aerobics are just two ways for them to keep their aerobic fitness up without fear of inducing asthma attacks.

General goals of asthma management include preserving normal lung function, minimizing symptoms and exacerbations, preserving physical fitness, and preventing mortality. These goals can be realized through physical activity and exercise, and patient and family education. Educational topics of particular importance for asthmatic patients are listed in figure 7.2. Comprehensive pulmonary rehabilitation programs with exercise training, education, and psychosocial intervention are ideally suited to meet these needs,[17-19] especially

---

Figure 7.2 Pulmonary Rehabilitation Program Modifications for Patients With Asthma

Exercise Assessment
Cardiopulmonary exercise testing (CPET) when possible
Evaluate for exercise-induced bronchoconstriction (EIB)

Exercise Training
Preexercise warm-up and postexercise cooldown
Premedication prior to exercise to prevent EIB
Upper and lower extremity strength and endurance exercise

Age-Appropriate Patient (and Family) Education
Recognition and avoidance of triggers
Role of medical therapy
  • Disease-modifying versus symptom-controlling medications
  • Importance of medication compliance
Peak expiratory flow monitoring
Variable symptoms of an asthma exacerbation
When to contact your care provider: developing an effective communicative relationship
Self-management plan
  • Management of baseline symptoms
  • Management of exacerbations
  • Stress, anxiety, and coping techniques
Dietary evaluation for patients requiring chronic systemic steroids

---

for patients with impaired pulmonary function or persistent symptoms who have functional disability despite standard medical treatment.

Supervised exercise training programs (such as pulmonary rehabilitation) improve the exercise tolerance of children and adults with asthma.[15,20-22] Aerobic fitness training using swimming,[15,23] walking, stair climbing, jogging, cycling,[20] rowing, and aerobics[21] have all been successful, and some cross-training benefits can occur.[15] Like other people, individuals with asthma can realize the following benefits from endurance training:

- Improved cardiopulmonary fitness with increased maximal oxygen consumption ($\dot{V}O_2$max)
- Delayed anaerobic threshold
- Reduced minute ventilation for a given submaximal work load

Similar to individuals without respiratory diseases, patients with asthma can increase their exercise capacity by following high-intensity training (e.g., at 50% to 80% of baseline $\dot{V}O_2$max or maximal heart rate).[15,20-24] Gains in exercise tolerance tend to be greatest in people with lower baseline fitness level.[15,25] Strength training is also of benefit. Other documented benefits of pulmonary rehabilitation for asthmatics include reduced asthma symptoms,[26] decreased breathlessness and anxiety during exercise,[15,20] decreased rescue beta-agonist use,[25,27] and fewer emergency department visits following, as compared with prior to, pulmonary rehabilitation.[26] There is no clear evidence to date that exercise training or pulmonary rehabilitation decrease bronchial hyperresponsiveness[20,23,28] or exercise-induced bronchoconstriction.[11,20,25] Further information is needed on the effects of pulmonary rehabilitation on quality of life for people with asthma.

A preexercise warm-up program and administration of inhaled beta-agonist is recommended for all asthmatics in pulmonary rehabilitation prior to exercise to decrease the likelihood of exercise-induced bronchoconstriction. Overall, the mode, intensity, and duration of exercise training should be individualized to meet the ability and needs of the patient, according to available resources. Incorporation of an exercise mode that is of particular interest to the patient may improve long-term maintenance of the exercise routine in the community setting. In patients with well-controlled asthma, the training intensity may be set near the anaerobic threshold or at a high percentage (i.e., 50% to 80%) of the maximal heart rate or $\dot{V}O_2$max, as determined by cardiopulmonary exercise testing. Low-intensity exercise, isometric exercise, or both, may be suitable for severely disabled people unable to exercise at higher intensity. Endurance training of the upper and lower extremities can promote weight loss and possibly reverse some of the muscle weakness caused by chronic steroid use. Because obesity (resulting from inactivity or chronic or frequent systemic corticosteroid administration) can also contribute to functional limitation, dietary intake should be evaluated and nutritional counseling provided to such people.

Whereas patients with mild asthma whose exercise tolerance is not impaired may benefit from the educational components of pulmonary rehabilitation, they may not require formal supervised exercise training. Comprehensive pulmonary rehabilitation is recommended for those asthmatics who are chronically ill with recurrent symptoms and functional limitations and disability despite optimal medical therapy. Recommended education topics, components, and program content to emphasize during pulmonary rehabilitation for patients with asthma are summarized in figure 7.2.

Cystic Fibrosis

Cystic fibrosis (CF) is an autosomal recessive inherited disorder in which abnormal epithelial ion transport leads to excessively thick, viscous mucus in the airways and impairs the secretion of pancreatic enzymes.[29-32] Consequences of these disturbances include recurrent respiratory tract infection with diffuse bronchiectasis, severe airflow obstruction, and hyperinflation. Similarly to patients with COPD, patients with CF experience recurrent exacerbations of disease characterized by increased sputum production, bronchoconstriction, and increased functional disability.[31-33] Patients with moderate to advanced disease may also experience intermittent hemoptysis, and often require periodic hospitalization. Severe nutritional impairment from inadequate dietary protein and fat absorption results from functional pancreatic insufficiency. The respiratory manifestations of CF typically begin in infancy or early childhood. Severe derangement of pulmonary function may be present by adolescence. Advances in medical management of CF have led to improved survival such that many patients live into adulthood.[29,34] Nevertheless, CF leads to major morbidity with symptoms of cough, sputum production, dyspnea, exercise intolerance, functional impairment, and impaired quality of life.[31,33] Patients often miss work or school and have difficulty participating in social or recreational activities because of frequent exacerbations (which may require hospitalization) especially in later stages of the disease. More than 90% of CF mortality relates to lung involvement.

Given the relative youth of CF patients, exercise responses tend to be normal until patients have moderate to severe disease.[35] Exercise tolerance is extremely variable among CF patients and is most limited at times of (or following) exacerbation. Following are factors that contribute to the exercise impairment of patients with CF:[31,33,36]

- Airflow obstruction
- Abnormal respiratory mechanics as a result of hyperinflation
- The need for increased total ventilation to overcome excess dead space and gas exchange disturbances

- Nutritional abnormalities
- Skeletal muscle dysfunction (related to deconditioning, reduction in muscle mass, alteration in fiber type, steroid treatment)

Patients with moderate to severe CF have ventilatory limitation to exercise (low breathing reserve with reduced $\dot{V}O_2$max and peak work rate).[33,36] Resting and/or exertional hypoxemia is common in later stages of the disease, and some patients may be affected by exercise-induced bronchospasm.[36] As in patients with COPD, leg fatigue or discomfort may be the major symptom limiting exercise for some patients with CF.[35] The cardiovascular response to exercise is normal in mild disease, but right ventricular (RV) stroke volume may be impaired once pulmonary hypertension develops in advanced disease.[32,33,35,36] Moreover, some patients develop hypertrophic osteopathy, which may diminish joint flexibility. Reduced physical activity can lead to greater difficulty clearing secretions. Aerobic fitness is an important prognostic feature for patients with CF because increased aerobic fitness is associated with improved survival and well-being.[32,36-38] Following are recommended medical treatments for CF:[39]

- Regular chest physical therapy with postural drainage to clear secretions
- Inhaled DNase to decrease mucus viscosity
- Antibiotic therapy for intercurrent infection
- Bronchodilators or intermittent steroid therapy
- Pancreatic enzyme and vitamin supplementation
- Maintenance of adequate nutritional intake
- Regular exercise

Lung transplantation is considered for patients with severe functional impairment and poor functional status. Interestingly, few CF specialty centers offer structured exercise programs.

Based on these considerations, pulmonary rehabilitation should be included routinely in the management of patients with moderate to severe CF. Exercise training and rehabilitation are highly beneficial, and clinical trials of exercise training have been reviewed.[33,40] Most studies have evaluated outcomes of training for adolescents and young adults. Exercise training for patients with CF leads to the following:[31-33,40-44]

- Improvements in aerobic fitness and endurance
- Increased strength

- Decreased breathlessness for submaximal tasks
- Improved quality of life

Enhanced sputum expectoration related to physical training (in conjunction with chest physical therapy) may account for the improvements in pulmonary function noted following exercise training in some studies.[33,41] Physical training alone should not, however, be considered a replacement for conventional postural drainage therapy. Maintenance of stable pulmonary function (i.e., prevention of decline) and exercise tolerance is crucial for patients with CF to prevent long-term worsening disability. The long-term effects of pulmonary rehabilitation on functional status, quality of life, frequency of exacerbations, hospitalizations, prognosis, and survival are not yet known in the CF population.

Although pulmonary rehabilitation for patients with CF shares many features that target patients with COPD, there are some important unique considerations for this patient population. Exercise tolerance cannot be predicted from resting measures of pulmonary function in CF patients.[45] Cardiopulmonary exercise testing is recommended at baseline to identify the precise factors contributing to exercise intolerance. Pulmonary rehabilitation professionals should instead assess the relative contributions of ventilatory limitation and deconditioning and make note of any cardiovascular limitation, assess the exercise level at which lactic acidosis occurs, and identify any exercise-induced bronchoconstriction or oxygen desaturation (and the level of exercise at which this occurs) to formulate a safe, effective aerobic training regimen for CF patients.[32,33,35,36,46]

The overall goals of exercise training in patients with CF are to maintain and optimize leg and arm function and minimize decline in strength, endurance, or functional capacity over time. Supervised exercise training should be undertaken for at least 20 to 30 minutes, 3 to 5 days per week for 12 to 16 weeks.[31,33,35,36] The intensity of training must be tailored to disease severity and patient tolerance. It is generally recommended that training be undertaken at moderate intensity (e.g., 50% of maximum work rate or 65% to 85% of the patient's individual maximal heart rate) as determined by cardiopulmonary exercise testing[35,36] for medically stable patients. Patients unable to exercise at this level may start at a lesser intensity or duration and increase exercise as they are able (e.g., by 10% to 15% or a few minutes each week) as the program progresses.[33,35,36] The intensity of training may need to be adjusted following disease exacerbations. Symptom-limited exercise may be appropriate for patients with more severe disease. Warm-up and cool-down periods should be provided. When possible, the exercise program should be tailored to include activities that the patient enjoys because motivation is important in promoting adherence to exercise over the long term.[33]

Ventilatory muscle training (resistive or threshold, conducted 10 to 30 minutes per day for several weeks) can increase inspiratory muscle strength and endurance in patients with CF.[47,48] The effect of ventilatory muscle training on overall endurance is inconsistent, but increased walking endurance has been noted in some patients.[49] Patients' oxygen saturation must be monitored and supplemental oxygen titrated to keep the S_aO_2 >88% because decreased tissue oxygen delivery may be harmful[46] and supplemental oxygen can improve exercise capacity and decrease dyspnea for hypoxemic patients.[31,32] CF patients with FEV_1 <50% or DLCO <65% predicted are most likely to desaturate with exercise.[36]

Patients and staff members must pay rigorous attention to hygiene techniques during rehabilitation to avoid cross-infection of patients with bacterial pathogens that may be antibiotic resistant.[41] Cross-infection of antibiotic-resistant organisms among CF patients is an extremely serious consideration that may alter the course of disease. Close attention must be paid to hand washing, universal precautions, and hospital-based aseptic techniques. Patients with CF should exercise at least three feet apart from one another and other patients in the program, and consideration should be given as to whether the CF patient should wear a protective mask.

Nutritional intervention is crucial to maintain growth and restore and maintain weight in CF patients.[50-52] Caloric and protein intake must be adjusted to meet the increased demand posed by exercise training.[53] Importantly, patients with CF have excess salt and fluid loss during exercise as a result of excessive sweating,[32,33] yet they may not experience thirst and tend to underestimate their fluid needs.[32,36] Therefore, close attention must be paid to maintenance of adequate fluid and salt intake.[32,35] Sport drinks can be useful both to replete electrolytes and provide caloric support.[42] Educational topics of particular importance to the CF patient include the following:

- Pacing
- Energy conservation
- Pursed-lip breathing
- Strategies to remain active in work, school, social, recreational, and sport activities
- The role of antibiotics and other medications (such as steroids and bronchodilators) in managing infection and optimizing lung function.

The rationale, importance, and techniques of chest drainage should be reinforced in CF patients. They should be instructed that although mechanical devices (e.g., vibration vest and positive pressure breathing devices) can assist secretion clearance, they should

---

Figure 7.3 Pulmonary Rehabilitation Program Modifications for Patients With Cystic Fibrosis

Exercise Assessment
Cardiopulmonary exercise testing
Identification of any exercise-induced bronchospasm (EIB)

Exercise Training
Warm-up and cool-down periods
Strength and endurance training: upper and lower extremity
Sodium chloride and fluid replacement especially when exercising in heat
Monitoring of oxygen saturation; maintaining S_aO_2 >90%

Nutritional Evaluation and Counseling
Weight monitoring during training

Age-Specific Patient and Family Education
Basis of symptoms (cough, sputum production, and dyspnea)
Medical therapy (antibiotics, bronchodilators, corticosteroids, vitamins, pancreatic enzymes, DNase)
Secretion clearance techniques
- Controlled cough
- Postural drainage
- Vibration vest and positive end-expiratory devices
- Bronchodilators
Pacing and energy conservation techniques
Pursed-lip breathing
Strategies to remain active in school, work, and recreational activities
Benefits of long-term maintenance of regular exercise
Potential role for lung transplantation in long-term disease management plan
Age-appropriate outcomes measures for exercise tolerance, dyspnea, and health status

not be substituted fully for manual chest physical therapy. Close partnering with health care providers and maintenance of regular long-term exercise are additional topics that should be addressed.

Finally, whereas some outcomes measures used for COPD such as the 6-minute walk test, cardiopulmonary exercise testing, shuttle walk test, and measures of dyspnea are also appropriate for patients with CF, the choice of health status tools needs to be tailored to the age and concerns of the CF patient. Tools that address well-being, self-worth, and physical appearance and perceived competence at school, with friends, in athletics, and in romance, such as the Quality of Well-Being Scale, the Self-Perception Profile for Children,[36,42] and the Beck Depression Scale, may be particularly useful outcomes measures for patients with CF. Figure 7.3 shows a summary of the issues to address in a pulmonary rehabilitation program for patients with cystic fibrosis.

Interstitial Lung Disease

Chronic interstitial lung disease is a heterogeneous group of disorders characterized by vari-able degrees of inflammation and/or fibrosis in the interstitial and/or alveolar compartments of the lung parenchyma. Examples of interstitial lung disease (ILD) are listed in figure 7.4 along with suggestions for exercise training and education topics. Typical symptoms common to most chronic forms of ILD include gradually progressive dyspnea on exertion and dry cough, with progressive exercise intolerance and fatigue.[54-56] In contrast to COPD wherein the principal respiratory derangements are airflow obstruction and lung hyperinflation, ILD typically manifests as a restrictive ventilatory defect, with low lung volumes and reduced diffusing capacity. Patients with ILD tend to have rapid, shallow breathing as a result of these alterations in respiratory mechanics. ILD patients experience impaired health-related quality of life related to the disease itself or its treatment.[57-59] In addition to dyspnea, patients with ILD typically have decreased peak oxygen consumption, maximal work rate, and endurance as compared to healthy people.[60-62]

The basis of exercise intolerance in ILD is multifactorial.[60-65] Airspace destruction or filling with inflammatory or fibrotic material leads to increased

---

Figure 7.4 Forms of Interstitial Lung Disease and Suggestions for Pulmonary Rehabilitation

Examples of ILD
Idiopathic pulmonary fibrosis
Sarcoidosis
Occupational lung disease (asbestosis, silicosis, pneumoconiosis)
Hypersensitivity pneumonitis
Drug-induced lung disease
Pneumonitis associated with collagen vascular disease
Adult respiratory distress syndrome (ARDS)
Bronchiolitis obliterans organizing pneumonia

Exercise Training
Strength and endurance training of the upper and lower extremities
Strong focus on pacing and energy conservation techniques
Assessment of oxygen requirements
 • Resting arterial blood gas
 • Exercise oximetry: test at highest intensity level to be performed using the patient's own portable system
 • High F_IO_2 may be required during exercise training
Nutrition counseling and prevention of muscle or weight loss

Education Topics
Nature and expected course of disease
Physiologic basis of symptoms and exercise limitation (emphasize that cough is not a contagious condition)
Expected benefits versus potential adverse effects of medical therapy
Rationale for and proper use of supplemental oxygen
Pulmonary drainage techniques (especially for persons with bronchiectasis)
Recognition of symptoms and signs of secondary infection
Prevention strategies: influenza and pneumovax vaccines
Community resources
Advance directives
Coping techniques for assistance in managing anxiety and depression
Training in options for and outcomes of mechanical ventilation

lung stiffness (reduced compliance), excess dead space ventilation, and impaired gas exchange. Because inspiratory capacity is impaired, the respiratory rate increases out of proportion to tidal volume during exercise. Hypoxemia may be mild at rest until advanced stages of disease, but exercise-induced oxygen desaturation is a hallmark feature of ILD. Expiratory flow limitation has also been reported in some people with ILD.[62] Any or all of these processes can lead to an increased work of breathing and ventilatory impairment to exercise. Concomitantly, alveolar capillary destruction (especially in patients with severe disease) may lead to further worsening of hypoxemia and increased pulmonary vascular resistance. Hypoxemia leads to both increased myocardial work and increased demand for a higher cardiac output, as well as decreased oxygen delivery to exercising muscles. Increases in pulmonary vascular resistance and pulmonary artery pressure can further impair cardiac function by impeding venous return to the left ventricle and can lead to exertional dizziness or syncope. Thus the patient with advanced ILD often experiences both circulatory and ventilatory limitation to exercise.

As is true of patients with other chronic respiratory conditions, patients with ILD commonly suffer from weight loss, reduction in muscle mass, and deconditioning.[61] Indeed, some patients report leg fatigue as the main reason for stopping exercise.[62] Because steroids are a prominent component of the medical treatment of some forms of ILD, steroid myopathy is also a particular concern in these patients.[57] Unlike the fixed structural abnormalities in the lung, the skeletal muscle dysfunction may improve as a result of participation in a pulmonary rehabilitation program.[8,66,67]

Many forms of ILD are progressive over time, with severely disabling symptoms, yet medical treatment options are often limited. In turn, many patients experience anxiety, hopelessness and depression, and embarrassment about their persistent cough. Selected people with advanced disease may be candidates for lung transplantation, yet this too is a major physical and psychological undertaking. Pulmonary rehabilitation is ideally suited to meet several of the needs of patients with ILD, and it is typically mandatory in preparation for lung transplantation.[68,69]

Supervised exercise training is useful to maintain or improve conditioning and possibly assist in recovery from steroid-induced myopathy. Patients with pulmonary fibrosis can achieve improvements in walking distance comparable to those made by patients with COPD following pulmonary rehabilitation.[69] Ideally, patients should be referred to pulmonary rehabilitation initially in the mild to moderate stage of disease, before they develop severe ventilatory limitation to exercise or severe pulmonary hypertension. As always, the exercise program should be tailored to meet the abilities and needs of the individual patient. Varying the intensity of exercise may be tolerated, depending on the nature and severity of the disease, comorbid conditions, and the severity of dyspnea.[70] General goals are to increase strength, endurance, and functional capacity (individualized to the interests, activities, and hobbies of the patient) and in turn to improve quality of life.

Exercise oxygen desaturation can pose a particular challenge to training, particularly among patients with advanced disease, because some patients desaturate profoundly (<88%) despite high-flow supplemental oxygen delivered via nasal cannula or oxygen reservoir device. Some patients with severe disease may even require a nonrebreather oxygen mask during exercise to maintain adequate oxygen saturation. Transtracheal delivery of oxygen is an alternate strategy to be considered for some patients. Maintenance of adequate oxygenation increases oxygen delivery to working muscles (including the heart) and can delay anaerobic threshold and in turn reduce the ventilatory requirement and improve $\dot{V}O_2$max.[71]

The patient's oxygen requirements should be assessed both by resting arterial blood gas testing and exercise oximetry. The oximetry should be performed at the highest intensity of exercises or activities the patient will perform in the program or in the home environment, using the muscle groups wherein the patient experiences the most dyspnea. This will ensure that oxygen supplementation is titrated adequately. Ideally patients should also be tested using the type of portable oxygen system they use outside the program because some systems (such as the pulse delivery of oxygen by electronic demand device) may not maintain adequate oxygen saturation during exercise in this patient population.

Because patients with ILD tend to have stiff lungs and high oxygen requirements, rehabilitation may not result in reductions in dyspnea. Patients should be taught pacing and energy conservation strategies as well as deep breathing techniques. An individualized plan should be formulated to enable each patient to continue participation in his or her individual hobbies and desired activities as long as possible.

The patient education topics recommended for inclusion in pulmonary rehabilitation for patients with ILD are shown in figure 7.4. Given the magnitude of disabling symptoms, and the progressive nature and poor long-term prognosis of some forms of ILD, particular emphasis must be placed on helping patients cope with anxiety and depression. Educational materials should also include a list of community services and resources. Importantly, pulmonary rehabilitation is an environment in which patients with ILD can become familiar with options for and outcomes of mechanical ventilation, and discussions can be held regarding advance directives and end-of-life care. Figure 7.4 lists disease types, exercise issues, and education topics appropriate for individuals with ILD.

Obesity-Related Respiratory Disorders

Obesity is a worldwide public health problem.[72-73] More than 50% of the adults in the United States are overweight or obese.[72,74] The medical morbidity associated with obesity accounts for a major component of national health care costs, and mortality is increased among obese people. Obesity is associated with numerous medical diseases, including diabetes mellitus, hypertension, cardiovascular disease (coronary artery disease and stroke), dyslipidemia, osteoarthritis, altered immune function, cancer, and gallstones.[72,75] Many of these disturbances have their onset during childhood or adolescence.[76] Importantly, several abnormalities of respiratory function can also result from obesity. People with "simple obesity" maintain a normal P_aCO_2 and have normal respiratory drive. In contrast, people with obesity hypoventilation syndrome (OHS) have daytime hypercapnia and hypoxemia, an impaired central respiratory drive with decreased ventilatory responsiveness to carbon dioxide and nocturnal hypoventilation.

Moderately to morbidly obese people, particularly those with OHS, typically have impaired respiratory system mechanics (with decreased lung volumes, decreased chest wall compliance as a result of the elastic load on the chest and abdomen, and decreased lung compliance resulting from the closure of dependent airways and the greater negative pleural pressure needed to initiate airflow), reduced respiratory muscle strength, or both.[77-79] Respiratory system resistance is simultaneously increased as a result of smaller airway caliber associated with decreased lung volumes. Larger airway resistance is typically normal. Patients with simple obesity may be relatively hypoxemic, but as noted, remain normocapnic. In contrast, people with OHS have daytime hypoxemia and hypercarbia, in part from a blunted respiratory drive. Such people often develop pulmonary hypertension, cor pulmonale, and respiratory failure. The hypoxemia results from a ventilation–perfusion mismatch and physiologic shunting through poorly ventilated alveoli at the poorly expanded bases of the lungs, as well as from overall hypoventilation. Collectively, these disturbances cause an increased work and oxygen cost of breathing.[77,78] Sleep-disordered breathing, including obstructive sleep apnea (OSA) and alveolar hypoventilation, are extremely common among obese people and can contribute to the development of pulmonary hypertension and cor pulmonale.[78,80] Moreover, obesity is associated with an increased risk of thromboembolic disease, aspiration, and complications of mechanical ventilation or anesthesia,[78] and poses difficulty or inability to perform several diagnostic tests.[75] Morbidly obese patients are at increased risk for developing overt respiratory failure.

Obesity is a major cause of dyspnea, exercise intolerance, functional limitation, disability, and impaired quality of life.[81-83] The following conditions impair exercise tolerance:[78,84,85]

- Pulmonary function and gas exchange derangements
- Increased metabolic rate relative to lean body mass
- High metabolic (oxygen) cost to perform modest exercise
- Circulatory impairment (claudication, microvascular disease, or both)
- Cardiac impairment (as a result of myocardial ischemia; pulmonary and/or systemic hypertension; and a hypervolemic, hyperdynamic state)
- Anxiety
- Deconditioning
- Mechanical inefficiency
- Musculoskeletal disturbances

Exercise limitation commmonly leads to a decreased ability to work or participate in recreational or social activities, difficulty performing activities of daily living (ADLs), and depression. Daytime somnolence resulting from sleep-disordered breathing can further impair neurocognitive and cardiorespiratory function. The coexistence of obesity and underlying lung or neuromuscular disease may increase impairments in pulmonary function and gas exchange and accordingly lead to worse disability.

Weight loss can lead to reductions in body fat,[86] improvements in lung function and gas exchange,[87-89] exercise tolerance and capacity,[78] and improvement of obstructive sleep apnea and sleep architecture.[90-91] It can also lead to improvements in cardiac function[92] and reductions of other medical complications. Dietary intervention, however, is commonly insufficient as a sole intervention to achieve significant weight loss, particularly for morbidly obese people. Successful weight loss often requires a combination of dietary intervention, behavioral modification, psychological support, and exercise. Some patients also require pharmacologic or surgical therapy.[93] Regular exercise is recommended by the American College of Sports Medicine[72] and the U.S. Centers for Disease Control and Prevention[94] as a crucial component of weight loss intervention programs. Exercise training, particularly in conjunction with caloric restriction, can lead to decreased body weight and fat, increased fat free mass, improvement in strength and endurance, and improved aerobic fitness.[72,95] Despite the recognized benefits and widespread recommendation for regular exercise, many obese people have difficulty initiating or adhering to a weight loss intervention, and few seek assistance from health care providers or participate in organized weight loss programs.[75] Importantly, very few traditional weight loss programs are configured to meet the needs of morbidly obese people or obese patients with pulmonary function or gas exchange impairments or respiratory failure.

Pulmonary rehabilitation is ideally suited to meet the needs of obese patients because of its ability to provide exercise training and recommendations for a long-term exercise program, extensive education, dietary counseling, and psychological support for anxiety and depression, while monitoring the patient's respiratory status closely. Inpatient programs may be particularly beneficial at the outset for people with low functional status (e.g., after a hospitalization for respiratory failure); complex skin care, personal hygiene, or other nursing needs; tenuous gas exchange; or a need for assisted nocturnal ventilation (CPAP or BiPAP). Goals of pulmonary rehabilitation for obese people with respiratory impairment include the following:

- Increased exercise tolerance (strength, endurance, or both)
- Improved gas exchange

- Weight loss
- Improved partnering between patient and health care providers through enhanced medical stability and increased knowledge
- Decreased disability and return to ADLs, hobbies, and work
- Acclimatization to and/or optimization of use of CPAP or BiPAP (with resultant improved sleep quality, gas exchange, daytime cognition, and mood)
- Assessment of needs for assistive equipment related to mobility, self-care, and hygiene
- Arrangement of home assistive services
- Education of the patient regarding additional outpatient resources

Pulmonary rehabilitation may be particularly useful as an intervention strategy for adolescents and young adults, to begin the process of change toward a healthier lifestyle. Patients with previously unrecognized obstructive sleep apnea can also be assessed, and recommendations can be made for polysomnography when appropriate. Indeed, comprehensive rehabilitation can lead to lower body weight and improved functional status and quality of life for obese people.[96-99]

When possible, cardiopulmonary exercise testing, pulmonary function testing, and assessment of gas exchange (and, where indicated, polysomnography) should be performed on obese people to identify the precise factors contributing to functional limitation prior to the initiation of pulmonary rehabilitation. If exercise testing is not feasible, consideration should be given to pharmacologic stress testing prior to exercise training to exclude untreated myocardial ischemia as a factor contributing to dyspnea. Consultation with a cardiologist may be necessary to assist in formulating the exercise prescription for some people. Oxygen saturation, pulse, and blood pressure should be monitored closely during exercise training. Educational sessions should focus on dietary counseling and the health benefits of weight loss, the rationale for and benefits of CPAP and BiPAP, anxiety management, coping strategies, and energy conservation strategies, as well as available community resources.

Additional special considerations apply to the rehabilitation of people with morbid obesity and people with severe obesity with concomitant lower extremity musculoskeletal disturbances. In general, rehabilitation of such people requires special equipment that can accommodate people of extreme weight. Morbidly obese people may not be able

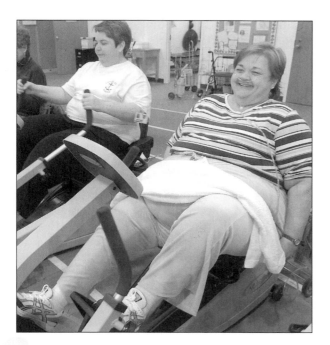

Proper exercise equipment is important for patients with obesity. Pulmonary rehabilitation facilities should have the right equipment to support all patients.

> ### Figure 7.5 Pulmonary Rehabilitation Program Modifications for Patients With Obesity-Related Respiratory Disease
>
> **Exercise Assessment**
> Cardiopulmonary exercise testing (CPET) where possible
> Consider pharmacologic stress testing, cardiology consultation, or both prior to program enrollment when CPET not done
>
> **Exercise Training**
> Strength and endurance training of lower and upper extremity muscles
> Walking and low-impact or water-based exercise for severely obese patients
> Staff familiarity with weight limits of program exercise equipment is crucial
> Bariatric assistive equipment (walkers, quad canes, scales, and exercise equipment) may be needed
> Consider need for extra staff to assist selected patients with transfers, stair climbing, etc.
> Wide, armless chairs that can accommodate persons of increased weight should be available
> Close monitoring for musculoskeletal problems
> Pacing and energy conservation techniques
>
> **Education Topics**
> Proper dietary choices
> Health benefits of weight loss and regular exercise
> Anxiety management and coping strategies
> Sleep-disordered breathing
> Detrimental health effects
> Rationale for and benefits of CPAP/BiPAP
> Community resources

to use standard exercise equipment such as cycle ergometers and treadmills. Staff members must be familiar with the weight limits of the equipment in their program. Walking, low-impact aerobics, and water-based activities are suitable forms of aerobic exercise for these patients. Recumbent bicycles, bariatric walkers, quad canes, commodes, wheelchairs, lifts, scales, and beds specially designed for obese people are commercially available. Extra staff may be needed to assist the morbidly obese patient with ambulation, transfers, stair climbing, and bed mobility.[98] Wide, armless chairs that can accommodate extra weight should be available. Collectively, the equipment and staff resources needed to serve obese people can lead to increased program costs, yet these costs are relatively small compared with the health care costs of untreated obesity and respiratory failure. Special considerations for pulmonary rehabilitation for patients with obesity-related respiratory impairment are shown in figure 7.5.

Pulmonary Hypertension

Normally, the pulmonary circulation is a highly elastic, high-capacitance system of blood vessels that can accommodate large increases in blood flow without an increase in pulmonary artery (PA) pressure. As such, under normal conditions, the increase in cardiac output associated with exercise (or the increase in blood flow to the contralateral lung following pneumonectomy) does not lead to increased PA pressure. Pulmonary hypertension (HTN) is present when the mean PA pressure exceeds 25 mmHg at rest or 30 mmHg during exertion.[100,101]

Pulmonary HTN can arise as a consequence of processes affecting the pulmonary vascular bed directly, or it may occur in conjunction with several respiratory or systemic diseases. Primary pulmonary HTN is a disorder wherein the pulmonary vasculature is affected in the absence of identifiable risk factors or coexisting disease. Common causes of secondary pulmonary HTN include advanced parenchymal lung disease (such as COPD or ILD), thromboembolic disease, HIV infection, collagen vascular disease (especially scleroderma or CREST syndrome), systemic-pulmonary shunts, left ventricular (LV) failure, drugs or toxins, sleep-disordered breathing (especially obesity hypoventilation), and pulmonary HTN associated with portal HTN/cirrhosis.[100,102] Pulmonary HTN is associated with a significant reduction in 5-year survival after diagnosis.

In both primary and secondary HTN, pulmonary vascular structural remodeling leads to increased pulmonary vascular resistance. In the presence of moderate to severe pulmonary HTN, PA pressure rises further when blood flow increases during exercise because vessels cannot be recruited or distended normally. Initially, the right ventricle (RV) compensates for the increased afterload by hypertrophy, dilatation, or both. Eventually, when the rise in pulmonary artery pressure or vascular resistance becomes too great, the RV can no longer maintain adequate forward flow, and cor pulmonale or circulatory collapse ensues. Hypoxemia (resulting from wasted ventilation, ventilation–perfusion mismatch, and/or right to left shunting), which is especially common during exercise or sleep, further increases PA pressure by causing hypoxic pulmonary vasoconstriction.[103] In situ thrombosis, typical in moderate to advanced disease, further worsens the pulmonary vascular resistance.

Exertional dyspnea, atypical chest pain, fatigue, palpitations, dizziness, and hemoptysis are characteristic symptoms of pulmonary HTN.[100] When severe, pulmonary HTN can lead to exercise-induced syncope, if the RV is unable to maintain forward flow to the LV, which in turn is unable to generate the cardiac output needed to meet the metabolic demands during exercise. The symptom of exercise-induced dizziness or presyncope is generally a sign of more severe disease and impaired RV function. Exercise intolerance (with low $\dot{V}O_2$max), early-onset lactic acidosis (i.e., at a relatively low work rate), and increased oxygen cost of work results from a combination of these cardiocirculatory and gas exchange impairments; secondary deconditioning also results from relative inactivity.[103] Patients with pulmonary HTN often have ventilatory limitation (with low breathing reserve), yet have demand for increased total ventilation to maintain effective alveolar ventilation and gas exchange.

Anticoagulation (to prevent in situ thrombosis) and supplemental oxygen (to maintain S_aO_2 >90%) with rest, exertion, and sleep are mainstays of medical therapy for pulmonary HTN.[100,102,104] People with P_aO_2 <55 mmHg at rest (or 55-59 mmHg with signs of RV dysfunction) or who have oxygen desaturation <88% during exercise are candidates for supplemental oxygen.[104] In addition, treatment with vaso-

dilators (calcium channel blockers or epoprostanol) or endothelin receptor antagonists is appropriate for patients with primary pulmonary HTN.[102,105] Although some patients with secondary pulmonary HTN are also candidates for vasodilator therapy (e.g., people with HIV or scleroderma), treatment of pulmonary HTN in these conditions is generally centered around treatment of the underlying disease.[102] Finally, lung (or heart–lung) transplantation is considered for some patients who have severe functional limitation and symptoms and an unfavorable hemodynamic profile and who have failed to respond to other treatment interventions.[102,105]

Until recently, pulmonary HTN was considered a contraindication for exercise training because of concerns of low cardiac output, arrhythmias, pulmonary venous congestion, and hypoxemia. However, the increased survival of patients on supplemental oxygen and medical therapy, the recognition that deconditioning is a coexisting factor contributing to exercise intolerance, and the inclusion of selected pulmonary HTN patients in lung transplantation programs has generated new interest in optimizing the functional status of these patients. Although exercise training and rehabilitation has not been shown (and is not expected) to improve PA pressure or cardiac output, it can lead to improvement in exercise tolerance by augmenting physical conditioning.[106] Pulmonary rehabilitation is currently undertaken as a routine part of pretransplantation preparation for these patients.

Several important special considerations do, however, apply to pulmonary rehabilitation and exercise training of patients with pulmonary HTN. Pulmonary rehabilitation should be closely supervised in a specialty center with staff who have experience treating these patients. Extreme caution must be undertaken to ensure that (1) the patient's medical treatment is optimized prior to referral for pulmonary rehabilitation and (2) that the patient and family understand the potential risks as well as benefits of exercise training. Frequent close communication with the patient's physician(s) and the pulmonary rehabilitation program medical director is mandatory during the program to ensure that the patient remains medically stable and that medical therapy remains optimized. Adjustments in anticoagulation, diuretic, vasodilator, and/or oxygen therapy may be necessary periodically. Decompensation of cor pulmonale with associated peripheral edema and/or pulmonary vascular congestion can worsen symptoms, gas exchange, or both, as well as further impair patient mobility.

Oxygen saturation should be monitored and oxygen titrated to maintain S_aO_2 >90%. Because of the potential for hypoxemia during exercise to further increase PA pressures and lead to arrythmias or circulatory collapse, it is reasonable to adjust the oxygen supplementation to achieve a higher S_aO_2 than would be considered usually necessary in the context of pulmonary rehabilitation for patients with other conditions.

Special safety precautions are necessary to prevent falls for anticoagulated patients with pulmonary HTN. Monitoring for any dizziness, palpitations or presyncope, systemic HTN, or hypotension is of paramount importance. To this end, high-intensity exercise, or any activities that could lead to increased intrathoracic pressure or decreased RV preload and precipitate circulatory collapse (such as weightlifting or other resistive exercises that require Valsalva effort) should be rigorously avoided. In general, low-intensity aerobic exercise (such as treadmill or level surface walking) is the mainstay of therapy. Telemetry monitoring may be necessary during exercise. Extreme caution must be undertaken to ensure that continuous intravenous vasodilator therapy is not interrupted.

HTN patients should be taught strategies for pacing and energy conservation, and some may benefit from assistive equipment for ADLs. Each patient must be assessed individually to understand the severity of the disease and the constellation of factors contributing to the exercise intolerance or functional limitation. Special considerations that must be heeded for patients with pulmonary HTN during pulmonary rehabilitation are shown in figure 7.6. Representative pulmonary rehabilitation exercise guidelines used by one specialty transplant center are shown in figure 7.7.

Figure 7.7 Exercise Protocol for Primary Pulmonary Hypertension Patients

1. No arm ergometry.
2. No resistive exercise (dumbbells, cuff weights, Cybex weight machines, Theraband).
3. Patients may perform floor exercise sitting in a chair. They do not get up and down off of the floor. They may perform active ROM with all extremities while participating in the floor exercise class.
4. PPH patients may use the stationary bicycle at no minimal resistance and may perform level surface track or treadmill walking.
5. May perform stretching exercises (i.e., hamstrings, heel cords, pulleys).

Reprinted with permission of Duke University.

Figure 7.6 Pulmonary Rehabilitation Program Modifications for Patients With Pulmonary Hypertension

Exercise Assessment
6-minute walk test
CPET

Exercise Training
Low-intensity aerobic exercise (treadmill or level surface walking)
Pacing and energy conservation
Avoid
- High-intensity exercise
- Activities that may lead to increased intrathoracic pressure such as weightlifting or resistive exercise that requires Valsalva effort
Telemetry monitoring for patients with known arrhythmia
Oxygen saturation monitoring:
- Supplemental oxygen to keep S_aO_2 >90%
- Ensure that patient's own portable system provides adequate S_aO_2
Close blood pressure and pulse monitoring during exercise
Stop exercise if patient develops chest pain, dizziness, lightheadedness, or palpitations

Higher intensity exercise may be considered post-transplantation

Crucial Additional Considerations
Close partnership between PR provider and patient's physicians needed
Avoid falls for anticoagulated patients
Ensure that continuous IV vasodilator therapy is not disrupted

Education Topics of Particular Importance
Anatomic and physiologic basis for symptoms resulting from pulmonary HTN
Signs of right heart failure
Importance and benefits of supplemental oxygen
Risks and benefits of anticoagulation
Vasodilator therapy
Lung transplantation
Mechanical ventilation
How to exercise safely to prevent deconditioning

Neuromuscular and Chest Wall Disorders

Some patients with neuromuscular or chest wall disease with respiratory impairment (with or without underlying lung disease) may benefit from pulmonary rehabilitation (see figure 7.8). The incidence, severity, and natural history of respiratory impairment in these disorders vary widely, but respiratory complications occur in the majority of people at some point in the illness. Many of these patients have concomitant skeletal muscle or joint dysfunction. The pathogenesis of the neuromuscular dysfunction and the respiratory disturbances in these individual disorders has been reviewed elsewhere.[107-113]

In brief, people with neuromuscular disease or restrictive chest wall disease tend to have restrictive ventilatory defects on pulmonary function testing with a rapid, shallow breathing pattern resulting from respiratory muscle weakness (or position-related mechanical disadvantage), or reduced chest

wall compliance (especially in people with kyphoscoliosis or Parkinson's disease). These abnormalities typically lead to gas exchange disturbances with elevated P_aCO_2 resulting from alveolar hypoventilation (particularly of the lung bases) and/or hypoxemia related to ventilation–perfusion mismatch or shunting (poor expansion of lung bases). The magnitude of derangement in gas exchange depends on the severity of illness.

The noted respiratory disturbances and concomitant peripheral muscle dysfunction in patients with neuromuscular or restrictive chest wall disease usually lead to exercise intolerance. Exertional dyspnea may be directly related to either respiratory muscle weakness or fatigue or the increased oxygen consumption that results from peripheral muscle weakness and general incoordination.[114] People with impaired expiratory muscle function also typically have a weak, impaired cough. Secretion clearance may be compromised further by poor lung expansion and chest wall distortion. Some patients, especially those with degenerative neu-

---

Figure 7.8 Pulmonary Rehabilitation Program Modifications for Patients With Neuromuscular and Chest Wall Disorders

Examples of Conditions Wherein Pulmonary Rehabilitation May Be of Benefit
Muscular dystrophy
Parkinson's disease
Multiple sclerosis
Postpolio syndrome
Myasthenia gravis
Restrictive chest wall disease (e.g., kyphoscoliosis, pneumoplasty)
Amyotrophic lateral sclerosis
Neuromuscular disease (including stroke) and comorbid primary lung disease

Exercise Training
Nature and goals of training program should be individualized to the following:
- Disease type and severity
- Individual patient needs and functional limitations
Avoid excess muscle fatigue
Consider consultation with neurologist or physiatrist in formulating exercise prescription (appropriate type and intensity of exercise)
Aerobic and strength training: ambulation, cycling, water-based exercise
More frequent, shorter duration exercise sessions may be needed
Interval training may be beneficial for some

Consider inspiratory muscle training in selected patients

Additional Considerations
Supplemental oxygen to keep S_aO_2 >88%
Potential role for noninvasive assisted ventilation during exercise
Identify patients who may be in need of nocturnal noninvasive assisted ventilation (CPAP or BiPAP)
Identify need for assistive or orthotic equipment to maintain independence with ADLs
Inpatient PR may be ideal for patients with severe functional limitation or intensive nursing or medical care needs

Educational Topics
Respiratory manifestations or complications of neuromuscular or chest wall disease (tailored to the individual's condition)
Secretion clearance and cough techniques
Recognizing signs of disease destabilization and infection
Rationale for and benefits of noninvasive assisted ventilation
Supplemental oxygen
Tracheostomy and mechanical ventilation
Advance directives
Community resources, skilled nursing facilities, chronic ventilator facilities

romuscular disorders such as muscular dystrophy, amyotrophic lateral sclerosis (ALS), multiple sclerosis, and Parkinson's disease, develop swallowing dysfunction related to pharyngeal muscle weakness or dyssynchrony and are at risk of aspiration. Collectively, all of these disturbances increase the risk of respiratory infection. Sleep-disordered breathing, including OSA and the worsening of alveolar hypoventilation during sleep, are very common among people with neuromuscular and restrictive chest wall disorders, especially in the advanced stages of disease.

Unfortunately, pharmacologic therapy for many forms of neuromuscular or restrictive chest wall disease is limited, and the conditions are often inexorably progressive and can lead to premature death. Medical complications and functional disability related to these disorders lead to significant health care costs, as well as to considerable stress, anxiety, and depression for the patient and family members. Supportive care, with emphasis on prevention of medical complications and maintenance of functional status, is therefore the principal focus of care.

Although very little data exists regarding outcomes of pulmonary rehabilitation for patients with neuromuscular or restrictive chest wall disease, programs can benefit such patients if the goals of intervention are appropriately individualized and tailored.[7,115-122] As such, the precise components included in the pulmonary rehabilitation program may differ from the typical program configuration geared toward the COPD patient. As in COPD, exercise training is undertaken in an effort to prevent or reverse deconditioning. However, particular caution must be undertaken to avoid excess muscle fatigue for people with degenerative neuromuscular disease or postpolio syndrome. People with significant skeletal muscle dysfunction may benefit in particular from water-based aerobic exercise. To date, no clear published guidelines exist regarding optimal exercise strategies for people with the different forms of neuromuscular disease, and further investigation is needed in this area.

When designing rehabilitation programs for these patients, the severity of the disease needs to be assessed. Consultation with the patient's neurologist or a physiatrist may be helpful in formulating a safe and appropriate exercise prescription. Strength training is usually included, but exercises may vary from resistive training to passive range of motion. Ambulation and cycle exercise can be performed by patients who have responded to medical therapy or are in an early stage of disease. More frequent

exercise sessions of shorter duration (interval training) may be used to avoid overstressing the patient's already limited neuromuscular status. Nocturnal, intermittent, or continuous mechanical ventilation may be needed for patients in advanced stages of disease.[123] Other interventions that may be helpful include the use of orthotics, postural drainage therapy, and inspiratory muscle training.[124-126] In addition to aerobic conditioning to maintain mobility and reverse deconditioning, identification and delivery of the adaptive equipment or orthotics needed to maintain independence with ADLs, work, driving, or attending school are particularly important aspects of pulmonary rehabilitation for this patient population.

Close attention should be given to training the patient in energy conservation and pacing techniques. Vocational rehabilitation may be useful for selected patients. Family members should be taught the basis of the patient's functional limitations and the optimal ways to provide assistance. As is true for interstitial lung disease, pursed-lip breathing training may not be appropriate for all people with neuromuscular disease. Oxygen saturation should be monitored during exercise, and supplemental oxygen titrated to achieve S_aO_2 >88%.

The pulmonary rehabilitation specialist should inquire whether the patient has been evaluated for or has documented sleep-disordered breathing. Non-invasive positive pressure ventilation (NIPPV) such as BiPAP can improve gas exchange disturbances, daytime respiratory function, and endurance and may lead to improved patient cognition as a result of improved sleep quality and prevention of nocturnal desaturation.[127,128] As such, an educational focus on the rationale for and benefits of nocturnal assisted ventilation, and assistance in acclimatization to this therapy in the context of pulmonary rehabilitation (especially inpatient pulmonary rehabilitation) can be extremely beneficial. In turn, patients may achieve further improvements in daytime function. NIPPV may also play a role in assisting patients' ventilation during exercise.

Inpatient pulmonary rehabilitation is particularly suited to the needs of these patients, particularly when severe illness and impaired functional capacity precludes participation in an outpatient pulmonary rehabilitation program. Inpatient pulmonary rehabilitation may also offer the opportunity to combine pulmonary rehabilitation with general neuromuscular disease–focused rehabilitation.

Patients should also be taught strategies to assist with cough and secretion clearance such as the manually assisted cough technique.[128] An insufflator–exsufflator device, vibration vest, or positive expiratory pressure device can be used where appropriate. Patients should be taught to identify early signs of respiratory infection and develop a clear process of communication with the health care provider to decide on a treatment strategy. Discussion of advance directives, mechanical ventilation, tracheostomy, home and community resources, and skilled nursing or chronic ventilator facilities is useful for some people to assist in evaluating their options for care should they develop progressive disease that renders them unable to remain at home. The principles and focus of rehabilitation specific to selected neuromuscular disorders are summarized in figure 7.8.

Lung Volume Reduction Surgery

Lung volume reduction surgery (LVRS) is a procedure wherein severely emphysematous lung tissue is resected via open sternotomy or video-assisted thoracoscopy in an effort to improve pulmonary function, respiratory mechanics, and exercise tolerance for highly selected patients with severe emphysema. Those who experience debilitating dyspnea and exercise intolerance despite optimal medical therapy and who are otherwise medically stable may be candidates. The surgical techniques, details of patient selection, and clinical outcomes have been reviewed.[129-132] Improvements in FEV_1, lung volume, gas exchange, exercise tolerance, dyspnea, and quality of life have been demonstrated following LVRS.[130,133-137] Clinical benefits tend to deteriorate within one to two years postoperatively, but some patients are improved for up to five years.[134] The noted benefits result at least in part from improved elastic recoil,[138] reduced hyperinflation and improved respiratory muscle function,[130,139,140] improved cardiac function,[141] and reduced central respiratory drive.[142]

The long-term survival, duration, and magnitude of the clinical benefits of LVRS were studied recently in the United States in the context of the National Emphysema Treatment Trial, a multicenter, randomized trial of medical therapy versus medical therapy plus LVRS for the treatment of patients with severe bilateral emphysema.[132,143] Results from this trial suggested that some patients, particularly those with FEV_1 <20% predicted value, and either diffusing capacity for carbon monoxide <20% predicted or homogeneous distribution of emphysema, are at higher risk of death following LVRS, and caution should be undertaken to avoid LVRS in these

patients.[144] People with upper lobe–predominant emphysema and baseline low exercise capacity following preoperative pulmonary rehabilitation gained a survival benefit at 24 months from LVRS compared to those in the medical therapy group.[143] Changes in exercise capacity, timed walking distance, quality of life, pulmonary function, and dyspnea at 6, 12, and 24 months were also greater in the surgery group. Additional research is needed to clarify the long-term efficacy of LVRS and to distinguish the patients who are most likely to benefit from those who are likely to have poor outcomes.

Some small, early lung cancers can be resected successfully during LVRS if they lie within the tissue targeted for surgical removal. The LVRS procedure has thus enabled surgical resection of early lung cancers for many patients who historically would have been considered inoperable because of the severity of their pulmonary function impairment.

Although the precise role of pulmonary rehabilitation in LVRS has not been defined clearly,[131] most experts agree that patients should only be considered for surgical therapy if they remain symptomatic despite maximal medical therapy and pulmonary rehabilitation.[132] In fact, assessments done during pulmonary rehabilitation may be of great value in determining the selection of the surgical candidate. In one study, patients with preoperative shuttle walk distances <150 meters had a greater risk of death.[133] Also, some patients who participate in a rehabilitation program may experience enough improvement to postpone or cancel surgery. Moreover, exercise training and pulmonary rehabilitation may potentially reduce some of the postoperative complications, and postoperative training may hasten recovery. It is unclear if preoperative improvement in exercise tolerance in pulmonary rehabilitation leads to postoperative mortality benefit. Thus the short-term benefits of LVRS compared to intensive medical therapy and pulmonary rehabilitation are not fully clear. One randomized, controlled trial did demonstrate greater improvements in lung function, gas exchange, 6-minute walk distance, and quality of life following pulmonary rehabilitation and LVRS compared with pulmonary rehabilitation alone.[145] More recently, the National Emphysema Treatment Trial reported greater increases in exercise capacity following pulmonary rehabilitation and LVRS compared with pulmonary rehabilitation and medical therapy alone among highly selected patient populations.[143] Exercise capacity improved by more than 10 watts in 16% of patients who underwent the surgery as compared to 3% of patients in the medical therapy group. These benefits were noted only among those people whose emphysema was predominantly upper lobe in distribution.

For patients who do undergo LVRS, good communication between the pulmonary rehabilitation program and referring pulmonary and surgical physicians is crucial for optimal results. The rehabilitation team should be familiar with the patients' goals, as well as the exercise training regimen (modes, intensity, and duration) recommended by the pulmonary and surgical team. A specific exercise prescription is usually formulated based on the results of comprehensive cardiopulmonary exercise testing. Following LVRS, pulmonary rehabilitation is helpful in reversing deconditioning, improving mobility, and monitoring oxygenation and the need for medications. The precise medical and training regimens needed may vary as the patient improves in the postoperative period. Pulmonary rehabilitation is the ideal setting in which to monitor patients for medical complications such as infection or ventilatory dysfunction. Early recognition can lead to prevention of more serious setbacks. The pulmonary rehabilitation program may need to be adjusted to accommodate thoracostomy tubes (necessary for the management of prolonged air leaks),

---

Figure 7.9 **Pulmonary Rehabilitation Program Modifications for Patients Undergoing Lung Volume Reduction Surgery**

PR assessments to help determine the selection of surgical candidates
Communication between pulmonary rehabilitation and surgical team
Preoperative exercise training to reduce postoperative complications
- Formulate exercise prescription based on CPET

Education
- Risks versus benefits of surgery
- Lung expansion techniques and mobilization postoperatively
- Pain management

Nutritional support
Postoperative exercise training
- Adjusted training regimen: increased intensity and duration over time
- Modification of immediate postoperative rehabilitation as a result of the following:
  Prolonged air leaks
  Extended tube thoracostomy
    - Concurrent medical conditions that precluded transplantation

---

assisted ventilation, or other medical complications. Aspects of pulmonary rehabilitation that require special consideration for patients undergoing LVRS are shown in figure 7.9.

Lung Transplantation

Numerous advances have been made in the immunobiology of organ transplantation in the past several years. Improvements in surgical technique, immunosuppressive therapy, and pre- and postoperative care have enabled patients with several forms of advanced respiratory disease to undergo lung or heart–lung transplantation. Other organs are occasionally also transplanted at the time of lung transplantation, and pulmonary rehabilitation specialists must remain alert to issues related to such procedures. International guidelines for the selection of lung transplant candidates have been published.[146] Overall survival rates are 60% and 65% and 40% and 45% at 2 years and 5 years, respectively.[146,147] Most transplant recipients experience significant improvements in exercise tolerance and quality of life.[148] Donor organ availability is limited, and patients may have to wait 2 or more years to receive a donor lung. Patients within accepted age guidelines[146] who have advanced emphysema (caused by smoking or alpha-1 antitrypsin deficiency), pulmonary hypertension, idiopathic pulmonary fibrosis (or fibrosis related to quiescent systemic disease), cystic fibrosis, or cardiopulmonary vascular disease wherein no further medical therapy is available and expected survival is limited may be considered for lung transplantation.[146,148,149] Absolute and relative contraindications for lung transplantation have been reviewed.[146,149] The underlying disease must be taken into consideration in determining proper pre- and postoperative medical management.[147] Disease-specific approaches in transplantation have been developed.[146,147,149] Pulmonary rehabilitation plays an essential role in the management of all patients both before and after lung transplantation.[150] Patients may require repeated rehabilitation if they require a repeat transplantation. Conditions for pulmonary rehabilitation of particular relevance to patients undergoing transplantation are shown in figure 7.10.

Before Transplantation

The primary goal of pretransplant rehabilitation is to optimize and maintain the patient's functional status while continuing close monitoring of the underlying disease.[151] Even patients with severe respiratory impairment may experience a reduction in dyspnea and an improvement in functional status.[152,153]

Figure 7.10 Pulmonary Rehabilitation Program Modifications for Patients Undergoing Lung Transplantation

Pretransplant
Disease-specific approach to exercise training
- Exercise intensity as tolerated by dyspnea, leg discomfort, and cardiorespiratory status
- Exercise intensity generally less than post-transplantation training
- Stable patient may exercise at home
- Periodic review of home exercise program and maintenance of exercise
- Maintain S_aO_2 >90%

Education
- Risks versus benefits of transplantation
- Potential complications
- Postoperative care
- Benefits and adverse effects of immunosuppressive medications
- Lung expansion and secretion clearance techniques
- Nutrition
- Methods of assisted ventilation
- Anxiety management, coping, and relaxation techniques

Identify patient and family expectations from transplantation

Immediate Posttransplant Period
Optimized airway clearance and lung expansion
Monitoring of changing requirements for supplemental oxygen

Improved stability in erect posture
Range of motion, basic transfer activities
Breathing pattern efficiency
Upper and lower extremity strengthening
Functional mobility and stable gait
Postural drainage and directed cough techniques
Analgesia titrated to exercise
Special walker to facilitate walking with chest tubes

Postdischarge
Exercise training
- Strength and endurance training of lower and upper extremities
- Continue oxygen saturation monitoring
- Emphasize postural awareness and breathing efficiency
- Back protection
- Increase intensity and duration of exercise over time
- Assess need for assistive devices

Educational topics
- Back protection
- Symptoms and signs of infection or rejection (including decreased exercise tolerance)
- Purpose and potential adverse effects of immunosuppressive therapy
- Maintenance of proper nutrition
- Importance of maintaining regular exercise

However, gains made in pulmonary rehabilitation do not usually eliminate the need for transplantation. It is possible that pretransplant pulmonary rehabilitation may decrease the risk of perioperative pulmonary complications and even decrease the duration of hospitalization after transplant.[150,151,153] A disease-specific approach to rehabilitation should be undertaken, as emphasized throughout this book (see disease-specific sections). Some modifications, however, may need to be considered.

Patients who are awaiting lung transplantation are typically those with the most severe underlying pulmonary disease. As a result, the intensity of exercise training may need to be reduced. Interval training (alternating brief periods of high- and low-intensity exercise) may be beneficial. Patients should exercise close to the highest work load they can tolerate from the standpoint of dyspnea or leg fatigue.[154] Exercise should be supervised to ensure that the prescribed work load can be safely tolerated but is intense enough to have a beneficial effect.

The patient must maintain the intensity of exercise achieved in pulmonary rehabilitation up to the time of surgery, preferably by undertaking exercise in a pulmonary rehabilitation center complemented by home-based exercise. Alternately, patients may require repeated intermittent admissions to pulmonary rehabilitation, and at least should maintain close contact with the pulmonary rehabilitation staff. The waiting time between transplant listing and actual surgery varies between 6 months and 2 years. During the time the patient is waiting for a transplant, the disease can progress, requiring reassessment and modifications in the patient's exercise program, medications, and oxygen prescription. Ongoing attendance in a pulmonary rehabilitation maintenance exercise program and periodic review of the home exercise prescription allow the pulmonary rehabilitation team frequent opportunities for reassessment and may also improve compliance and minimize the severity of pretransplant medical complications. Pulmonary rehabilitation is an ideal setting in which to educate the patient and family regarding the following:

- Expectations from surgery and the perioperative period
- Potential complications of transplantation
- Benefits and side effects of immunosuppressive agents
- Lung expansion and secretion clearance techniques
- Methods of assisted ventilation
- Strategies to optimize nutrition

After Transplantation

Postoperative rehabilitation can begin as early as 24 to 48 hours after surgery. The goals of rehabilitation in this phase include optimizing airway clearance and lung expansion postextubation, decreasing the requirements for supplemental oxygen, and improving stability in the erect posture.[155] Patients may experience tingling or pain in their extremities while their body adjusts to the immunosuppressive medication. Rehabilitation in this early period should include range of motion, basic transfer activities (e.g., sitting to standing), breathing pattern efficiency, upper and lower extremity strengthening, functional mobility (e.g., ambulation), and postural drainage therapy. Directed coughing is especially important because of the impairment in the cough reflex that results from denervation of the donor lung.

Resistive exercise of the upper and lower extremities can be performed in addition to simple ambulation. Special walkers can be used to facilitate walking while chest tubes are still in place. Analgesia needs to be titrated so exercise can be performed without worsening incisional pain. Poor posture can also result from incisional discomfort. Pain may be relieved by medications, heat or ice, massage, and transcutaneous electrical nerve stimulation (TENS). The chosen pain management strategy should be implemented in conjunction with the patient's physician. When surgery has been performed via a median sternotomy or antero-lateral thoracotomy, adequate time (i.e., 4 to 6 weeks) should be allowed before the patient can engage in strenuous upper extremity exercises such as arm cycling and wall pulley weights.

Prior to discharge, it is important to check that the patient's gait is stable (i.e., the patient is at low risk for falls) and that lower extremity strength is adequate (i.e., for such tasks as transferring into and out of bed or chairs or climbing stairs). Oxygen saturation should be monitored during different levels of exertion so that patients and their families are aware of oxygen requirements during ADLs and exercise at home. Specific assistive medical equipment should be given where necessary.

After discharge from the hospital, patients may return to the rehabilitation program site for additional training and evaluation of exercise tolerance. Postural awareness, maintenance of good posture and back protection measures, avoiding rotation, and flexion, need to be addressed to prevent spinal compression

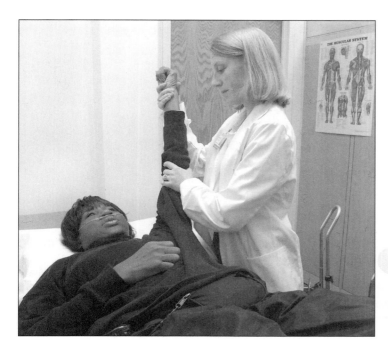

Lung transplant patients should begin postoperative rehabilitation immediately, within 24 to 36 hours after the transplant. Basic skills such as sitting, standing, and walking, as well as range of motion skills, should be emphasized.

fractures secondary to osteoporosis as a result of the prolonged use of immunosuppressive medications. The major goal of rehabilitation during this phase is to achieve increased tolerance for activities of daily living as well as close medical monitoring.

Patients often have difficulty performing a symptom-limited maximal exercise test shortly after discharge. The 6-minute walk test is simpler to perform and can usually be completed by the patient prior to resuming outpatient rehabilitation. Serial repetition of these tests at regular intervals (e.g., 3, 6, or 12 months after transplant) can be helpful in following the patient's progress; a decrease in exercise tolerance may be an early indicator of infection or rejection. On the other hand, patients may be able to exercise at progressively higher intensity, duration, or both following uncomplicated lung transplant because they are no longer primarily ventilatory limited. Patients may need reassurance that they can safely perform activities that are more strenuous than those performed prior to transplant. It may be helpful to follow parameters that reflect functional status such as the 6-minute walk test and maximum $\dot{V}O_2$max measured during a pulmonary exercise stress test.[156-158] Pulmonary rehabilitation staff must also be aware that musculoskeletal problems may arise once the patient is exercising at a higher intensity or duration level.

Another long-term goal is to attenuate the cardiovascular effects (hypertension and hyperlipidemia) and steroid-induced muscle dysfunction associated with long-term immunosuppressive therapy.[159] Further work is needed to clarify the effects of exercise or pulmonary rehabilitation on morbidity and long-term survival following transplantation. Posttransplantation education should focus on the following:

- Maintenance of regular exercise
- Proper nutrition
- Recognition of symptoms and signs of infection or organ rejection
- Long-term adverse effects of immunosuppression such as neuropathy, gait disturbances, or osteoporosis

Lung Cancer and Thoracoabdominal Surgery

Lung cancer is the leading cause of cancer deaths among men and women in the United States and elsewhere in the developed world.[160] Cigarette smoking is the major cause of lung cancer,[161] and women are more susceptible to tobacco carcinogens than men.[162] Asbestos and other environmental exposures, including passive smoke exposure, are other etiologic factors. Lung cancer contributes substantially to health care costs, and 5-year survival is only ~14%. Many patients with lung cancer, including those recovering from radiation or chemotherapy, are excellent candidates for pulmonary rehabilitation especially given that they may also have COPD. Once they are medically stable, such people should undergo a program of pulmonary rehabilitation to improve their functional status and quality of life.

Surgical resection is the treatment of choice for non-small-cell lung cancer that is detected at an early stage.[163,164] For some patients with lung cancer, attempt at curative resection requires wedge resection or lobectomy; others require total pneumonectomy.

When considering pulmonary resection for a patient with chronic lung disease, medical personnel must assess whether the patient has adequate respiratory reserve to tolerate the intended surgery and to estimate the risk of postoperative complications. Similar concerns pertain to patients with respiratory disease who are facing open heart surgery such as coronary artery bypass or other thoracic or upper abdominal surgery. Screening spirometry is needed for all patients with chronic respiratory disease prior to thoracic or upper abdominal surgery. In general, any patient undergoing thoracic, upper abdominal, or abdominal aortic aneurysm surgery is at risk of developing postoperative pulmonary complications, particularly if the person has smoked within two months of surgery or has underlying chronic lung disease or poor general health status.[165] The following postoperative respiratory complications are major causes of perioperative morbidity and mortality:[166-169]

- Infection
- Atelectasis
- Worsened gas exchange
- Bronchoconstriction
- Thromboembolic disease
- Respiratory failure requiring prolonged mechanical ventilation

Patients with preoperative FEV_1 >2 L can generally tolerate pneumonectomy, and patients with baseline FEV_1 of 1 to 1.5 L can usually tolerate lobectomy. Postoperative predicted FEV_1 should be >0.8 to 1 L or >40% predicted.[170,171] Predicted postoperative diffusing capacity <40% is a risk factor for postoperative complications.[170,172]

Importantly, preoperative exercise tolerance is also a significant predictor of patients at risk for poor outcome following thoracotomy.[173-177] Comprehensive exercise testing may be useful in the preoperative assessment of patients whose pulmonary function criteria are borderline. Those people who achieve $\dot{V}O_2$max >15 ml/kg are likely to tolerate surgery, whereas those with $\dot{V}O_2$max <15 ml/kg are at higher risk of complications.[173,174] Stair climbing ability can also predict cardiorespiratory complications following lung resection surgery.[177]

As is true for patients undergoing lung transplantation, pulmonary rehabilitation can play an important role in optimizing the patient's medical and functional status prior to major thoracic or upper abdominal surgery, and can assist in preventing complications and restoring functional status postoperatively. The basic principles of pulmonary rehabilitation for pre- and postoperative rehabilitation for patients with lung cancer or others facing surgery are the same as those for patients not undergoing surgery. However, some specific considerations apply to the patient preparing for or recovering from surgery.

When possible (depending on the type of surgery), patients with advanced lung disease should undergo regional rather than general anesthesia. Also, where feasible (i.e., nonemergent surgery), patients should abstain from cigarette smoking for at least two months preoperatively.[178] Smoking cessation is an important part of preoperative pulmonary rehabilitation. Patients should be trained preoperatively in lung expansion and secretion clearance

techniques, including deep breathing, incentive spirometry, and assisted coughing.[167,179,180] Specific attention should be paid to the factors contributing to the patient's baseline functional impairments so as to design a successful program for the patient in the postoperative period. Patients should also be trained in pacing, energy conservation, pain management, and venous thrombosis prevention strategies, as well as in methods for performing transfers and bed mobility (to plan for the time when a thoracostomy tube is needed after surgery). Exercise capacity should be measured by cardiopulmonary exercise testing or a stair climbing test preoperatively, and a training regimen should be instituted in the weeks prior to surgery to improve strength and endurance. Actual training duration should be based on the time frame for surgery as dictated by medical necessity.

Postoperatively, patients should be mobilized as early as possible. Implementation of pain control and lung expansion strategies learned prior to surgery are crucial to minimize atelectasis and assist in the clearance of secretions in the early postoperative period. Gas exchange should be monitored closely, and noninvasive positive pressure ventilation (NIPPV) [such as bi-level positive airway pressure (BiPAP)] should be used as necessary if not contraindicated from a surgical standpoint or because of a risk of aspiration. Sputum analysis should be obtained and antibiotics started early for any signs of evolving bacterial respiratory infection. Adequate nutritional intake should be assured. Stretching, range of motion, and/or ambulation exercise should begin as soon as is medically feasible.

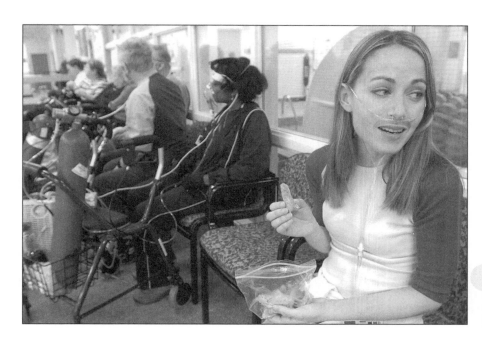

After surgery, patients should not just exercise but also keep up their energy through proper nutrition.

As for patients who have undergone lung transplantation, those who have had pulmonary resection or major abdominal surgery can continue training to improve strength and endurance in a standard outpatient pulmonary rehabilitation program following discharge from the hospital. Further studies are needed to assess the impact of pulmonary rehabilitation before and after lung resection or other thoracic surgery on perioperative complications and survival. A summary of the program content and components that need to be emphasized or modified for patients undergoing pulmonary resection or other thoracic or upper abdominal surgery is shown in figure 7.11.

Figure 7.11 Pulmonary Rehabilitation Program Modifications for Patients With Lung Cancer or Those Undergoing Thoracic or Upper Abdominal Surgery

Exercise training to increase muscle strength and endurance
Attend PR once chemotherapy or radiation therapy is completed
Self-management strategies
Assess need for assistive equipment and services
Psychosocial intervention: coping, stress, and anxiety management techniques
Education
- Breathing retraining
- Pacing
- Energy conservation
- Nutrition
- When to seek health care services

Mechanical Ventilation

Patients with severe lung disease that require mechanical ventilation at home may be candidates for pulmonary rehabilitation. Noninvasive mechanical ventilation also may be considered as an adjunct to exercise training.

Noninvasive Ventilation and Exercise Training

The reduced ventilatory capacity and dyspnea associated with chronic respiratory disease relate in part to the combination of increased elastic and resistive loads to breathing as well as mechanical disadvantage of the respiratory muscles resulting from dynamic hyperinflation, particularly in COPD.[181] Dynamic hyperinflation worsens during exercise because of the faster respiratory rate and associated reduced exhalation time. Similar problems commonly afflict people with CF. For some patients undergoing pulmonary rehabilitation, the severity of ventilatory limitation and dyspnea limits their ability to perform aerobic exercise. Although exercise duration and a sense of well-being can be improved by low-intensity exercise, high-intensity exercise is needed to achieve gains in the physiologic parameters of aerobic fitness.[182-184] People with severe hyperinflation, restrictive chest wall disease, or weak respiratory muscles often have difficulty training at higher intensity levels. As such, the potential role for NIPPV in improving exercise tolerance for patients with chronic respiratory disease has been investigated.

Continuous positive airway pressure (CPAP) has the potential to assist breathing during exercise by opposing the inspiratory threshold load to breathing that results from dynamic hyperinflation. Indeed, low levels of CPAP (up to 5 cm water) applied via face mask to patients with COPD[185-188] and severe CF[189] during submaximal exercise can relieve dyspnea, reduce inspiratory effort, and improve exercise duration. However, other studies have failed to demonstrate beneficial effects of CPAP during exercise and have cautioned that excess positive airway pressure may increase the expiratory work of breathing, hyperinflation, or both.[187]

Pressure support ventilation (PSV) is a mode of ventilation wherein pressure is applied during inspiration only. This can decrease the inspiratory work of breathing and enhance tidal volume while allowing the patient to set his or her own respiratory cycle.[190] Proportional assist ventilation (PAV) is a newer mode wherein the pressure delivered varies in proportion to the respiratory effort made by the patient.[191] This mode can provide ventilatory assistance with enhanced patient comfort.[187,191] These modes also have demonstrated success in improving exercise duration when delivered noninvasively via face mask,[185,187,191-194] reducing inspiratory effort and dyspnea[185,187,195] without the risk of worsening expiratory work of breathing for patients with COPD. PAV or PSV can also improve the pattern of breathing during exercise (increase tidal volume and decrease respiratory rate), improve gas exchange, and enable the COPD patient to achieve a higher work rate and reduce lactic acidosis during training.[196,197]

Although NIPPV is not yet used routinely in pulmonary rehabilitation, these findings render NIPPV a promising adjunct to exercise training in pulmonary rehabilitation for selected people. However, technical and logistic difficulties must be overcome to use NIPPV during exercise training; for example, potential benefits are overshadowed by the discomfort of wearing the face mask for some patients.[198] The use of nocturnal NIPPV in the home is an alternate strategy to enhance the benefits of exercise training for selected patients with COPD by providing respiratory muscle rest during the night.[199] The role for NIPPV in improving nocturnal alveolar hypoventilation, gas exchange, and daytime function for patients with respiratory dysfunction as a result of neuromuscular or chest wall disease is well established.[123,127,200] Few studies, however, have investigated NIPPV as an adjunct to exercise training for these people. Assist-control ventilation during exercise improved endurance and breathlessness for patients with sequelae of tuberculosis.[201] Further work is needed to clarify the role for NIPPV as an adjunct to pulmonary rehabilitation for patients with chronic respiratory disease. The optimal strategies for its use remain undefined, and it is unclear as yet whether improvements in exercise endurance or intensity achieved by exercising with NIPPV translate into overall improved functional status. As such, NIPPV is not currently recommended for routine use during pulmonary rehabilitation, but may be considered for selected patients with severe ventilatory limitation and hypercarbia who are extremely limited in exercise tolerance and gain relief of symptoms by exercising with mask ventilation.

Ventilator Dependency

An increasing number of patients with chronic respiratory failure are returning to their home environments while still receiving intermittent, continuous, or nocturnal ventilatory support.[202-206] These patients, who are often discharged after long stays in acute or extended care facilities, typically suffer from significant atrophy of the peripheral skeletal muscles. Critical illness, prolonged immobility, poor nutritional status, and corticosteroid and other medication usage may contribute to muscle weakness. Measures to improve peripheral muscle strength and endurance may increase patient independence and thus quality of life, and may free some patients from ventilatory assistance over the long term. Nutritional assessment is important for these patients to determine if supplementation (e.g., via feeding tube) is needed, which will also increase muscle strength and exercise tolerance.

Strength training can be accomplished by using free weights, gravity, manual resistance, and elastic bands, as well as other methods described in chapter 4. Some patients can undertake endurance training such as walking or cycle ergometry exercise while receiving mechanical ventilatory assistance under the supervision of a trained health care provider. Patients who receive intermittent ventilatory support may benefit from beginning training during periods of mechanical ventilation. Adjustments in ventilator settings, including the mode, tidal volume, respiratory rate or F_iO2, may be required. As strength and endurance improve, exercise training with the usual modalities during periods of spontaneous breathing may be added.

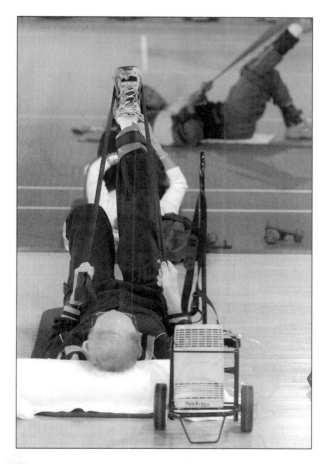

Even patients who require the use of oxygen or ventilators need to exercise. Light exercise such as lifting free weights and using elastic bands are good ways to keep up strength and enhance overall well-being.

Patients who require chronic tracheotomy placement have limitations in their speech and are at risk for swallowing dysfunction. Evaluation by a speech therapist can identify problems in these areas. The use of cuffless or fenestrated tracheotomy tubes or Passey Muir valves can allow for speech, and compensatory swallowing maneuvers can often prevent aspiration. See figure 7.12 for a list of the program content and components that need to be emphasized or modified for patients who are ventilator dependent.

Figure 7.12 Pulmonary Rehabilitation Program Modifications for Patients Who Are Ventilator Dependent

Age-specific patient and family training
Nutrition assessment
Strength training, walking exercise, or both
Intermittent ventilatory support
Exercise training during periods of mechanical ventilation
Adjustment in ventilator settings during exercise (e.g., F$_I$O$_2$) as needed
Speech therapist evaluation to facilitate patient communication

---

Pediatric Patients With Respiratory Disease

Children are commonly affected by respiratory disease, including many of the disorders discussed earlier in this chapter. However, a few additional considerations should be noted in the pediatric population. Of note, the prevalences of asthma and obesity are rising in children as well as adults. Also, children are increasingly among those under consideration for lung transplantation. Children with respiratory disorders are often kept from participating in athletic activities. Optimal medical therapy and preexercise warm-up routines can result in normal tolerance for athletic activities in children with asthma and other respiratory conditions. Family members, schoolteachers, coaches, and physical education teachers all require instruction regarding the importance of exercise and safety issues for children with respiratory disease. The benefits of regular exercise training have been dis-

cussed previously and apply to children as well. Care should be taken to ensure that the pulmonary rehabilitation program designed for children is interesting and fun. Figure 7.13 lists the program content and components that need to be modified for pediatric patients with respiratory disease.

Figure 7.13 Pulmonary Rehabilitation Program Modifications for Pediatric Patients With Respiratory Disease

Age-specific patient and family training
Optimal medical therapy for the underlying condition
Preexercise warm-up routines
Family members, schoolteachers, coaches, and physical education teachers instructed in the following:
  • Exercise and safety issues
  • Benefits of regular exercise training
  • Bronchodilator therapy
  • Postural drainage
  • Early treatment of respiratory tract infections
Recognition of the child in respiratory distress

Patients With Coexisting Respiratory and Cardiac Disease

The coexistence of cardiac disease with respiratory disease poses particular challenges to the PR specialist. Given that cigarette smoking is a common risk factor for both conditions, many people acquire both respiratory and cardiac disease (e.g., coronary artery disease and ischemic cardiomyopathy). Special consideration must be given to the educational, psychosocial, and exercise needs of such patients to determine whether pulmonary rehabilitation, cardiac rehabilitation, or both may be appropriate. To this end, the pulmonary rehabilitation provider and pulmonary rehabilitation program medical director should work closely with the patient's referring physician to do the following:

  • Identify the multifactorial basis of symptoms and functional limitations
  • Formulate a safe program of exercise training

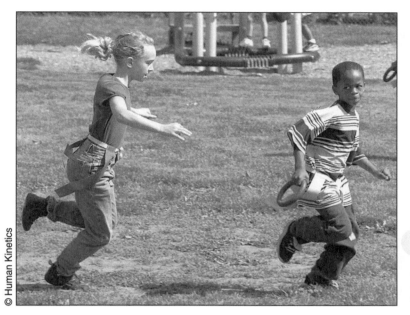

© Human Kinetics

Children with respiratory diseases should be encouraged to exercise. Teachers, coaches, and parents should encourage activity, but they also need to know the child's limits.

- Determine those aspects of a rehabilitation program that may help the patient the most

The choice of cardiac or pulmonary rehabilitation may depend on the predominant factors identified as contributing to exercise limitation during a cardiopulmonary exercise test, as well as physician or patient preference, insurance reimbursement, and local availability. Smoking cessation is a crucial topic to emphasize in both types of programs. An extensive discussion of cardiac rehabilitation is beyond the scope of this chapter, but has been reviewed elsewhere.[207-208]

In brief, although the precise program content varies, pulmonary and cardiac rehabilitation share many features, including the combination of exercise training, education, and psychosocial intervention. The goals of each are to improve or maintain functional independence, empower patients to gain control over and better cope with their symptoms and disease, and initiate behavioral modifications that help to prevent the worsening of disease over time. Skeletal muscle dysfunction contributes significantly to the exercise intolerance of patients with congestive heart failure[208] as well as that of people with COPD and other forms of chronic respiratory disease. Exercise training leads to improved exercise capacity, improved skeletal muscle function, reduced dyspnea and fatigue, and improved New York Heart Association Functional Class for people with congestive heart failure.[208] Cardiac rehabilitation is considered appropriate for patients with stable class II or III heart failure who do not have serious arrythmias or other contraindications to exercise such as unstable angina.[208] Thus, such patients who also have pulmonary disease may be candidates for pulmonary rehabilitation.

Patients with underlying cardiac disease and pulmonary disease participating in a pulmonary rehabilitation program may require telemetry monitoring. They should stop exercising if they develop chest pain; discomfort; a burning sensation, heaviness, or pressure in the chest, neck, jaw, or arms; dizziness; unusual shortness of breath; palpitations; or extreme fatigue. Such symptoms may prompt the need for further medical testing prior to the patient continuing in the program.

Increasingly, pulmonary rehabilitation and cardiac rehabilitation programs are combining rehabilitation for patients with mixed cardiac and respiratory disease into one program. The best way to integrate the principles and components of cardiac and pulmonary rehabilitation to optimize outcomes for people with combined disease is an area that merits further study.

Conclusion

Most of the experience in the field of pulmonary rehabilitation has been in working with patients with COPD. However, patients with other causes of chronic respiratory disease also benefit from pulmonary rehabilitation with improved respiratory symptoms, functional status, and tolerance of ADLs. Close evaluation of the patient's pathophysiology and good communication with the patient's primary care physician or pulmonologist will allow for an individually designed, disease-specific approach to pulmonary rehabilitation for these patients. Pulmonary rehabilitation professionals must expand their knowledge and understanding to help optimize life for patients with all types of respiratory disease.

chapter 8

Program Management

This chapter covers the basic principles of pulmonary rehabilitation services management, which include the structure of the interdisciplinary team, the team members' qualifications and responsibilities, and the administrative aspects of program management. The facility's needs, patient populations served, and available resources determine the structure of the team. Specific management areas to consider include the following:

- Program location
- Facility
- Group size
- Staffing ratios
- Program certification
- Equipment
- Time constraints
- Common types of pulmonary patients admitted to rehabilitation
- Adherence to the standards of the Joint Commission on Accreditation of Health Care Organizations (JCAHO)
- Health Insurance Portability and Privacy Act (HIPPA) standards

The program coordinator must be familiar with all areas of reimbursement and the importance of thorough documentation. Developing a marketing strategy and plan with the interdisciplinary team members is also a key ingredient in promoting awareness of the program. By applying the basic principles of management, success with pulmonary rehabilitation services can be achieved.

Medical Director

Pulmonary rehabilitation services must be provided under the direction of a licensed physician who has training or experience in the care of patients with chronic respiratory disease. The medical director is an integral part of the pulmonary rehabilitation team and supervises and guides each patient's plan of care. The medical director or physician designee is responsible for the safety and quality of care provided, provides direct supervision, and therefore has a high level of involvement with patients and staff. Although referrals may come from various physicians in the community, the medical director is ultimately responsible for determining the appropriateness of the pulmonary rehabilitation plan of care for the patient.

The medical director has many responsibilities. Medicare and Medicaid guidelines state that all reimbursable services in pulmonary rehabilitation are incident to physician services. Although this does not necessarily always require the continuous physical presence of a physician, a physician must be kept continually informed and assume an active role in all aspects of the pulmonary rehabilitation process. This must be documented in the rehabilitation medical record. For safety reasons, direct supervision by a physician—not necessarily the medical director—is a necessity. Documentation of daily physician supervision in the record is also necessary. "Incident to" language, as currently interpreted by the Office of the Inspector General, requires a physician to personally see the patient sufficiently often to evaluate the course of treatment and, when necessary, make adjustments to the treatment plan.

The medical director may function as clinician, administrator, educator, and advocate. Clinical responsibilities include providing expertise on the appropriateness of the referral, participating in the initial assessment and goal development, and reassessing the patient's progress and goals during the rehabilitation intervention. Physician input is important in identifying the medical factors contributing to exercise limitation. Pulmonary services must be tailored to the patient's individual needs. After an appropriate exercise evaluation and input from team members, the physician should be directly included with the exercise prescription and supervise the patient's care.

Physicians need not be continuously present in the immediate exercise area, but must commit to being available to evaluate patient needs and manage programmatic issues in a timely fashion. The physician in the rehabilitation setting has a unique opportunity to evaluate patients during exercise training over an extended period of time, thus enabling clinical observations not commonly possible in the office setting. Hypoxemia with ambulation, comorbidities such as cardiac or peripheral vascular disease, and orthopedic concerns may be uncovered as formerly sedentary patients begin to participate in exercise training. Clinical progress and concerns that evolve during rehabilitation can then be communicated to the referring physician.

Administrative involvement of the medical director includes review and approval of the mission statement, policies, protocols, and procedures. The medical director should review budgetary matters and attend administrative meetings to help monitor and direct program growth and development. Educational efforts should include conferences with patients, staff, and colleagues. Advocacy for pulmonary rehabilitation can raise public awareness as well as increase the visibility and understanding of this service in the medical community.

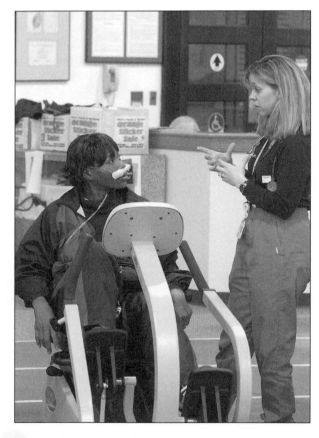

The medical director isn't responsible for only administrative tasks. The director also needs to work one on one with a patient to ensure adherence to the rehabilitation program.

Education of health care professionals, especially those in training, should be a prominent role of all members of the pulmonary rehabilitation team. The medical director should actively participate in this process. In particular, medical students, residents, and pulmonary fellows should be encouraged to take electives in pulmonary rehabilitation, under the direction of the medical director. This will enhance understanding of pulmonary rehabilitation and foster timely referrals among the medical community.

The medical director, along with the rehabilitation team, is ultimately responsible for services provided during pulmonary rehabilitation. Collaborative teamwork will ensure the best outcomes for patients.

Program Coordinator

The pulmonary rehabilitation program coordinator (sometimes also called the program director) plays a pivotal role in the rehabilitation team, serving as a liaison among the patient, medical director, referring health care providers, administrators, and other rehabilitation staff. The program coordinator or health care professional designee trained in pulmonary rehabilitation performs an initial entry assessment.

He or she provides or oversees the skilled pulmonary rehabilitation treatment directed toward patients' specific goals. The coordinator then refers the patient to appropriate interdisciplinary team members for discipline-specific evaluations. The coordinator has clinical, administrative, educational, and advocacy responsibilities and works in close collaboration with the medical director in all aspects of pulmonary rehabilitation services and management.

In view of these responsibilities, the Guidelines Committee of the AACVPR recommends that the program coordinator have graduated from an accredited school of a cardiorespiratory health–related field (e.g., physical therapy, respiratory therapy, nursing, exercise physiology, occupational therapy) and hold the national certification or licensure if appropriate for his or her health care profession. The Guidelines Committee also recommends that the program coordinator have a minimum of three years of clinical pulmonary rehabilitation experience following a bachelor's or higher degree, or at least five years of pulmonary rehabilitation experience following an associate's degree. The coordinator must have special training and experience in working with patients with pulmonary diseases and in the services delivered in pulmonary rehabilitation, and have advanced

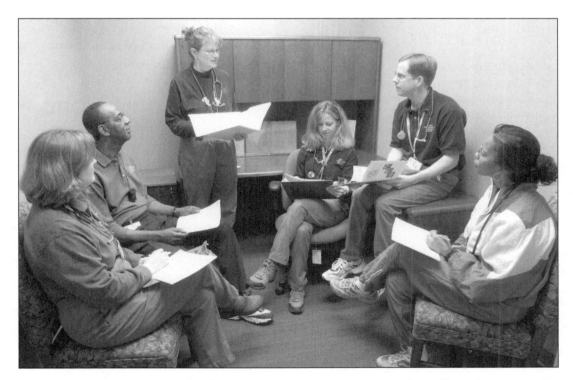

A good pulmonary rehabilitation program must have the right team members. These team members must work together, drawing on each other's knowledge and strengths, to provide the best services to their patients.

training and experience that allows him or her to meet the competencies described in appendix D. The program coordinator must have all the qualifications of the pulmonary rehabilitation specialist outlined in the following section.

Rehabilitation Specialist

The rehabilitation specialist must have formal education in a cardiorespiratory health care specialty (e.g., physical therapy, respiratory therapy, nursing, exercise physiology, occupational therapy, psychology, nutrition) and have special training and experience that allows him or her to meet the competencies described in appendix D. The rehabilitation specialist participates in the skilled, discipline-specific evaluations and ongoing treatment (e.g., exercise training, education, and psychosocial support) of the patient, under the direction of the program coordinator.

Rehabilitation specialists may come from diverse academic preparations and clinical experiences. The program coordinator and the medical director are responsible for structuring the pulmonary rehabilitation program to ensure optimal use of the rehabilitation specialist's expertise.

Interdisciplinary Team Structure

The interdisciplinary team structure consists of the medical director, program coordinator, rehabilitation specialist, and other professionals who provide specialized services (e.g., nutritionist, chaplain, pharmacist) for the respiratory patient. The structure of the interdisciplinary team depends on a number of factors, including the characteristics of the patient population, the program budget, reimbursement, and the availability of team members and resources. Because of program and staffing constraints, the program coordinator may also by necessity have to assume the role of the rehabilitation specialist.

Under the supervision of a licensed health care professional, team members may work full- or part-time, on call, or as consultants or volunteers. It is desirable to have at least one full-time team member, usually the program coordinator. Members of the team may include the following:

Chaplain or pastoral care associate

Clinical psychologist

Dietitian or nutritionist

Exercise physiologist

Home care personnel

Licensed counselor

Licensed vocational or practical nurse

Medical director

Occupational therapist

Patient

Pharmacist

Physiatrist

Physical therapist

Physician extender—PA, NP

Psychiatrist

Pulmonary fellows, residents, interns

Pulmonary laboratory technologist

Pulmonary rehabilitation specialist

Recreational therapist

Referring physician

Registered nurse

Rehabilitation coordinator

Rehabilitation program graduate

Respiratory therapist

Social worker

Speech therapist

Students—medical, physical therapy, nursing

Vocational rehabilitation counselor

Staff Competencies

Documentation of staff competencies must be performed regularly. This is usually under the direction of the program coordinator. Training the interdisciplinary team members to be rehabilitation specialists will require a consistent orientation program for all new staff members and an annual skills update and assessment. Examples of documentation include licensure renewals, CPR certification, and completing required JCAHO and HIPPA training sessions.

Core Staff Responsibilities

To achieve patient and program goals, the pulmonary rehabilitation team, consisting of the medical director, program coordinator, rehabilitation specialist, and interdisciplinary members, must have the knowledge, communication skills, and technical skills necessary to carry out the following responsibilities:

- Ensure patient safety
- Assess the patient
- Develop an individualized treatment plan with collaborative patient goals
- Document the need for a skilled level of care and services
- Conduct patient education and training sessions
- Evaluate patient progress
- Reassess the treatment plan
- Participate in pulmonary rehabilitation team conferences, staff meetings, and in-services, as appropriate
- Monitor patient outcomes
- Develop a home program plan to promote long-term adherence to recommended lifestyle changes
- Implement continuous quality improvement (CQI) and performance improvement principles
- Initiate departmental emergency procedures as necessary
- Provide in-services to other departments
- Recommend pulmonary rehabilitation to potential patients
- Serve as role models through their attitude, communication style, and professionalism
- Communicate with the referring health care physician to ensure that the patient is seen sufficiently often to assess the course of treatment and the patient's progress, and—when appropriate—to adjust the course of treatment

Every member of the pulmonary rehabilitation interdisciplinary team should assume the role of patient advocate, with a strong belief in and understanding of the goals of pulmonary rehabilitation. The number of team members and their professional backgrounds will vary considerably from one facility to another. It is not necessary for every member of an interdisciplinary team to assess each patient; however, the collective knowledge, skills, and clinical experiences of the team should reflect the interdisciplinary expertise necessary to achieve the desired patient and program goals and outcomes. Team communication and interaction are vital to the successful rehabilitation of the patient. Pulmonary rehabilitation professionals do not just treat the disease; they treat the patients as human beings, with empathy and compassion.

Continuing Education

Continuing education is necessary in the field of pulmonary rehabilitation to maintain a high level of expertise. Completion of continuing education units is often dictated by individual disciplines. Attendance at the annual national and state meetings of the AACVPR will meet many continuing education requirements. The Guidelines Committee recommends joining state or regional chapters of the AACVPR (if available) and participating in the annual meeting of this organization.

Minimum Staffing Requirements

During the initial or subsequent assessments, problems requiring the intervention of another skilled professional may be identified. Examples would be the identification of significant psychosocial dysfunction requiring the intervention of a skilled mental health professional, nutritional problems requiring a nutritionist, musculoskeletal problems requiring a physical therapist, or respiratory care procedures requiring a respiratory therapist. Under these circumstances, the need for these professional services must be ordered and clearly documented by the medical director or referring physician.

Staffing Ratios for Exercise

Pulmonary rehabilitation programs have a specific staffing framework with minimum requirements to support appropriate pulmonary rehabilitation services. Every program should have a medical director, a program coordinator, and at least one rehabilitation specialist. As stated earlier, in some programs the program coordinator may also serve as the primary rehabilitation specialist. Individual staff roles and responsibilities have been previously described.

Patients with chronic respiratory disease need close monitoring during exercise training as a result of changing hypoxemia, bronchospasm, dyspnea, chest pain, dysrhythmias, weakness, and comorbidities.

At a minimum, one pulmonary rehabilitation specialist per four exercising patients is reasonable. However, for patients with severe disease or

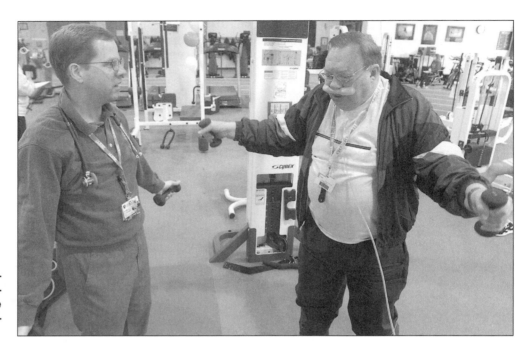

The proper staff-to-patient ratio is important to ensure the safety and well-being of patients.

substantial comorbidity, one-on-one staffing may be necessary.

Staffing Ratios for Education and Psychosocial Support

For instruction that permits individualized interactions, demonstrations, and skills practice, one pulmonary rehabilitation specialist can lecture to a classroom of eight patients.

Because of the complex nature of the disease and its comorbidity, specific patients may need one-on-one education on selected educational topics (e.g., breathing retraining, inhaler use, oxygen adjustments, and coughing and pulmonary hygiene techniques).

For didactic (generalized) educational lectures such as instruction on the anatomy of the lung, the class is not limited in size.

Because of the complex nature of impairment in psychological functioning, a patient with substantial comorbidity in this area should be referred to a mental health provider for further evaluation and treatment. The initial assessment will help identify the need for such a referral.

Program Components and Structure

Pulmonary rehabilitation services use a physician-directed interdisciplinary approach directed toward individualized patient goals. Services provided by various disciplines must be reasonable, medically necessary, and distinct from one another. Pulmonary diagnosis, special precautions, goals of treatment, frequency, and duration need to be clearly documented.

Initial Assessment and Goal Setting

The initial pulmonary rehabilitation assessment sets the foundation for all services provided during pulmonary rehabilitation. This assessment, which is described in chapter 2, is performed by the program coordinator or designee. The evaluation includes a review of the patient's medical history, current medical regimen, and comorbid conditions. The purpose of the assessment is to identify problems, establish short- and long-term goals in collaboration with the patient, and develop a comprehensive individualized plan of care. The plan of care must be approved by either the referring physician or the medical director. This process is time intensive and often takes up to 2 hours or more.

Education and Skills Training

The educational component of pulmonary rehabilitation, which is detailed in chapter 3, includes group lectures, small-group demonstrations, interactive sessions, and one-on-one sessions for specifically identified patient needs. Educational needs are determined during the initial evaluation and should be reassessed during the program. The objective is to train patients to achieve optimal levels of understanding and self-management through maximal function, transfer of gains to the home setting, long-term adherence, and a reduction in dependency. The program coordinator or rehabilitation specialist and other interdisciplinary team members with special training or expertise in a particular content area should present the relevant information at the education and skills training sessions. The entire educational process usually requires 24 hours over the course of the program.

Therapeutic Exercise

An individualized physical conditioning and exercise program using proper breathing techniques is essential for strength and endurance training to improve functional capabilities. Disease-specific approaches to exercise training are detailed in

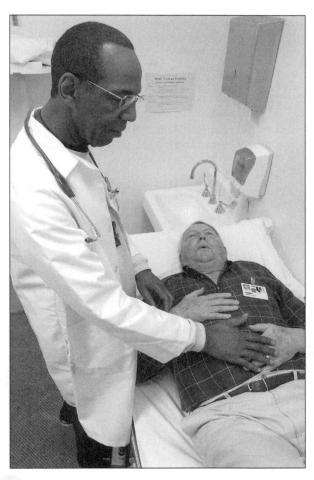

Breathing retraining is an important component of therapeutic exercise for the pulmonary patient.

chapters 4 and 7. To ensure the safety of patients with pulmonary disease, clinicians should address appropriate bronchodilation, adequate oxygenation, and optimal dyspnea management. Breathing retraining, energy conservation, and relaxation techniques are often taught in conjunction with exercise. Supervised exercise training is facilitated by the use of various types of equipment. The goal should also include the development of an exercise program that can be translated into the home environment and incorporated into the patient's activities of daily living (ADLs).

Clinicians must clearly document the rationale for continued skilled intervention for any exercise program. Because exercise without a documented need is not covered by insurance, clinicians must document progress toward specific goals, as well as examples of carryover to the home setting. The documentation should tell a progressive story from point A (initial assessment of problems) to point B (achievement of stated goals).

Exercise training in pulmonary rehabilitation usually requires 36 hours of supervised exercise to ensure that benefits are occurring, potential complications are addressed, and patients understand and are comfortable with exercise procedures so that long-term adherence occurs.

Psychosocial Services

The psychosocial component is critical to the success of pulmonary rehabilitation. Psychosocial support services are detailed in chapter 5. Problems such as depression and anxiety are common in patients with chronic respiratory disease and impair their function and ability to perform ADLs. Screening questionnaires are available to complement the psychosocial information obtained by assessment. Psychosocial intervention reinforces breathing retraining, relaxation, stress management, and panic control, which can be beneficial in reducing the anxiety/dyspnea cycle and should be an integral part of the overall treatment plan. Patients experiencing substantial impairments in psychological functioning should be referred to a mental health provider for further evaluation and treatment. Reassessment of psychological status and refinement of interventions is an essential component of discharge planning. Developing a plan for the maintenance of activities that promote and reinforce strategies learned will be useful in the long-term maintenance of physiologic and psychosocial gains. This intervention, offered in either individual or group formats, can also be effective in reducing distress and facilitating adaptive coping. Psychosocial intervention usually requires 10 hours of treatment within the pulmonary rehabilitation program.

Encouraging Adherence and Promoting Long-Term Gains

Strategies to improve long-term adherence with the principles taught and practiced during the formal pulmonary rehabilitation are essential to the maintenance of educational, functional, exercise performance, psychosocial, disease management, and health maintenance gains. These strategies optimally are incorporated into all aspects of the pulmonary rehabilitation process. Promotion of long-term adherence is discussed in chapter 5. Practical examples include teaching self-management strategies in the domiciliary setting, fostering lines of communication with health care providers, integrating principles of energy conservation into ordinary ADLs, formulating an exercise training plan for the nonrehabilitation setting such as the home or a local gymnasium, and encouraging participation in local support groups such as better breathing clubs. The patient should come to realize that the formal rehabilitation process is but a short component in a lifestyle change that should last a lifetime. A postrehabilitation exercise maintenance program for graduates would also foster adherence to the exercise prescription. Because these strategies promoting the long-term maintenance of gains are

ideally integrated into virtually every aspect of pulmonary rehabilitation (and indeed are necessary for optimal care), they do not, per se, require an additional time allotment.

Duration of Program

Generally, outpatient pulmonary rehabilitation requires up to 72 hours of participation. The specific program configuration depends on program goals, staff and space availability, and budgetary considerations. Examples of 2-days-, 3-days-, and 5-days-a-week pulmonary rehabilitation program schedules are given in appendix E. The program duration for each patient is ultimately determined by the accomplishment of his or her individual goals.

On occasion, certain medical circumstances may necessitate readmission to a pulmonary rehabilitation program. Patients with chronic lung disease are susceptible to periodic exacerbations or other complications that may significantly reduce their health status. For example, hospitalizations for exacerbations of the chronic disease, lung resection, transplantation, or lung volume reduction surgery may be valid reasons for readmission in a pulmonary rehabilitation program. Such reenrollment requires appropriate evaluation and documentation of medical necessity. Most patients reenrolling would not require the full complement of services; such limits should be determined on an individual basis.

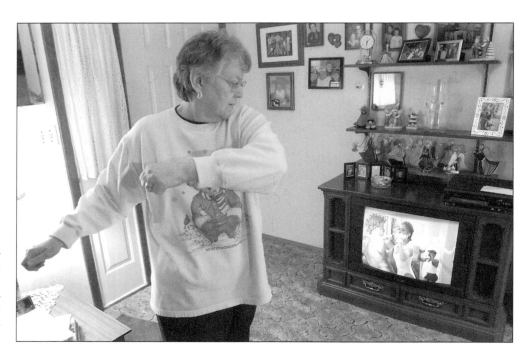

A good rehabilitation program will promote continued activity and well-being, even after formal rehabilitation is over.

Policies and Procedures

The pulmonary rehabilitation staff must be familiar with the policies and procedures of their department and facility. These may include the following:

- Mission statement
- Scope of care including location of services, hours of operation, content, description and schedule, patient selection criteria, and emergency procedures
- Staff requirements including job descriptions, responsibilities, in-service attendance, evaluations, and dress code
- Medical record documentation
- Continual quality improvement
- Patient's rights
- Administrative policies including patient's rights, organizational ethics, and management of information as mandated by HIPPA (privacy, confidentiality, security, record retention, availability of medical records)
- Infection surveillance and control
- Safety
- Facility orientation including confidentiality, payroll, security, employee benefits, and risk management

Facilities and Equipment

The facilities and equipment used for the pulmonary rehabilitation program should meet state, federal, and JCAHO safety code standards. Sufficient space should be available for the multiple services provided. The equipment budget should address equipment expenses in relation to purchase, maintenance, and depreciation. The physical area can vary greatly depending on program structure, patient population, needs, and resources. Because the program is often the first contact patients and the general public have with the health care facility that houses it, the program plays an important role in public relations for the entire organization. An organized, clean, and well-maintained facility provides patients with a sense of ownership and enhances patient satisfaction and safety. The following should be considered for the pulmonary rehabilitation space and equipment:

- Adequate and convenient parking, including handicapped parking spaces
- Access to the building for people with disabilities
- Easily accessible water or drinking source
- Rest rooms with handicap access
- Sufficient space for classroom, exercise, clinical, and administrative activities
- Oxygen source (e.g., piped in, liquid, concentrators, E-cylinder) and delivery systems
- Optimal light, temperature, ventilation, and humidity
- Strict avoidance of scented perfumes, deodorants, and hair sprays by staff and patients
- Storage space for equipment (oxygen, wheelchairs, walkers, respiratory therapy equipment) and locked medical records
- Hand washing facilities with antibacterial soap and waterless disinfectant
- ADL facilities such as a teaching kitchen, bed, washer and dryer, and tool bench to help train patients in their specific ADL needs
- Avoidance of chemical odors from cleaning agents, new paint, and whiteboard markers
- A copy of the Patient's Bill of Rights displayed in the department (see figure 8.1)
- Confidentiality of patient records and patient privacy
- First aid supplies
- Bronchodilator medications and nebulizer
- Resuscitative equipment, including a bag mask and a standard defibrillator or automatic external defibrillator (AED)

See appendix F for an example of a typical pulmonary rehabilitation facility.

Emergency Procedures

Appropriate emergency procedures and supplies must be available in the pulmonary rehabilitation exercise testing and training areas. The staff must be certified at least in basic life support and ongoing clinical competency demonstrations, including mock drills. All staff members should be familiar with the program's emergency policies and procedures. A standing order from the referring physician or the medical director for the rehabilitation program emergency procedures is needed. Minimum emergency equipment should include the following:

- Oxygen source and delivery apparatus
- Bag-valve mask device

Statement of Patient's Rights

Thank you for choosing our Pulmonary Rehabilitation Program for your outpatient rehabilitation needs. To receive the most out of your program, we want you to know the following information.

Your Rights

You have the right to:

- Exercise these rights without regard to sex, culture, economic, educational or religious background or the source of payments for your care.
- Receive considerate and respectful care at all times and under all circumstances, with the recognition of personal dignity.
- Know the name of the pulmonary rehabilitation program coordinator who has primary responsibility for coordinating your pulmonary rehabilitation program and the names and professional relationships of the interdisciplinary team members who will see you.
- Receive information about your illness, course and outcome of treatment in terms that you can understand.
- Receive as much information about the pulmonary rehabilitation program and the components that it entails so you can give informed consent or refuse this course of treatment.
- Participate actively in decisions regarding your care. This includes the right to refuse treatment.
- Full consideration of privacy when attending the pulmonary rehabilitation program. Some of the areas are not as private as we would like them to be. Let us know if you are not comfortable discussing issues with the team members in this setting. You have the right to be advised as to the reason for the presence of an individual.
- Confidential treatment of all communications and records pertaining to your care. You will need to provide written permission before medical records can be released.
- Reasonable responses to any reasonable requests you may make for service.
- Reasonable continuity of care and to know in advance the time and location of appointments as well as the identity of persons providing the care.
- Be advised of any research affecting your care. You have the right to refuse to participate in such research projects. Any experimental or research activities will require your informed consent.
- Be informed of any continuing health care requirements following your discharge from the pulmonary rehabilitation program.
- Examine and receive an explanation of your bill regardless of source of payment.
- Know that all patient rights apply to the person who may have legal responsibility to make decisions regarding medical care on your behalf.
- Wear appropriate personal clothing and religious or other symbolic items, if desired, as long as they do not interfere with diagnostic procedures or treatment.
- Expect reasonable safety insofar as the pulmonary rehabilitation program practices and environment are concerned.
- Discuss or resolve ethical issues surrounding your care.

Your Responsibilities

We ask you to assist us by:

- NOT wearing perfume, cologne, aftershave, or heavily scented lotions, as many patients are allergic to these products.
- Providing complete and accurate information regarding your medical history.
- Reporting changes in your condition to the pulmonary rehabilitation team members.
- Providing written consent for treatment as requested.
- Complying with your instructions and letting the pulmonary rehabilitation staff know when you are not able to.
- Asking questions of the pulmonary rehabilitation staff and participating in your care.
- Being considerate of others and respecting their confidentiality and privacy. Our space is not always as private as we would prefer. Please leave the information you may overhear or see here at our facility.
- Being on time or calling if you are unable to attend the pulmonary rehabilitation program as scheduled.
- Meeting financial responsibilities, including provision of appropriate insurance and billing information.

Figure 8.1 Patient's Bill of Rights.

Compliments and Concerns
- If you have a compliment regarding the pulmonary rehabilitation program or a specific team member, please share it with the staff and the pulmonary rehabilitation program coordinator. You may also want to write a letter to the facility administrator.
- Direct any concern or complaint regarding your treatment while in the pulmonary rehabilitation program to the program coordinator. If you do not feel your concern was adequately addressed or would prefer to speak to someone else, ask for _____ (the department facility manager). If you still do not feel your concern has been adequately addressed, contact the Quality Review Department at the facility. You have the right to expect a response within a reasonable time frame.

Figure 8.1 *(continued)*

- Oral airway
- Pulse oximeter
- First aid supplies
- Standard defibrillator or automatic external defibrillator (AED)
- Suction equipment (optional, for special patient requirements)
- Medications: nebulized bronchodilators and sublingual nitroglycerin

Pulmonary Rehabilitation Location: General Issues

Pulmonary rehabilitation can be conducted in inpatient, outpatient, home-based, or community-based settings. The focus of these guidelines is outpatient pulmonary rehabilitation, which is by far the most common in the United States. Important questions arise regarding the physical location of pulmonary rehabilitation programs, however. Although many outpatient programs are located within the four walls of the traditional acute care hospital, some are located in satellite facilities not in immediate proximity to the hospital. A number of comprehensive outpatient rehabilitation facilities (CORFs) also provide pulmonary rehabilitation. Additionally, a limited number of physicians' offices provide pulmonary rehabilitation. The consideration regarding physical location of a rehabilitation program is secondary to the absolute requirement that the program meet all the necessary standards regarding accessibility for the patient, safety, provision of services, adequate physical space, and availability of staff and physician resources.

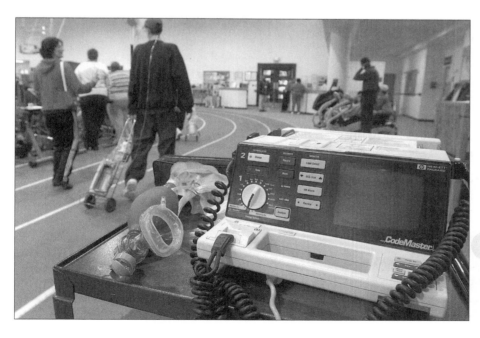

The health and safety of rehabilitation patients is vital. Proper emergency equipment must be easily accessible in all rehabilitation programs.

AACVPR Program Certification

The American Association of Cardiovascular and Pulmonary Rehabilitation (AACVPR) instituted program certification in 1998 to recognize programs that were meeting the published *Guidelines for Pulmonary Rehabilitation* and the *Guidelines for Cardiac Rehabilitation and Secondary Prevention*. These documents are regularly updated to reflect changes in the standard of care. Program requirements for certification generally follow the recommendations published in the guidelines. For information regarding program certification, the AACVPR can be contacted through its Web site, www.AACVPR.org.

The Guidelines Committee recommends that pulmonary rehabilitation programs document their adherence to nationally accepted standards through participation in a certification program such as the AACVPR accreditation program. This will provide for enhanced quality of pulmonary rehabilitation services. Furthermore, program certification may become a prerequisite for third-party reimbursement in the not-too-distant future.

Documentation

Accurate and thorough charting facilitates effective communication among the team, the referring physician, and third-party payers. Documentation is used to delineate the functional abnormalities of the patient and the clinical rationale for treatment, monitor patient progress, demonstrate outcomes, and provide CQI. Documentation is also a necessary precursor to reimbursement. It must reflect the need for professional supervision of the treatment, the level of skilled care, and progress toward rehabilitation goals.

Documentation Required for the Initial Referral to Pulmonary Rehabilitation

The physician's order for pulmonary rehabilitation must be present before the initiation of services. This must include the pulmonary diagnosis, the objectives of treatment, the frequency and duration of skilled services, and special precautions. Verbal orders must be cosigned, usually within 24 hours.

Documentation Required at the Initial Assessment

Documentation at the initial assessment is discussed in detail in chapter 2. This documentation should include the following:

- Physician's evaluation of the history of the respiratory illness and significant comorbidity
- Diagnostic tests relevant to the patient's specific pulmonary problems
- Symptom assessment, including levels of dyspnea and fatigue
- Level of pain
- Prior functional levels
- Specific problems and functional deficits in areas of exercise, gait, ADL performance, nutritional status, knowledge base, and psychosocial status
- Rehabilitation potential: poor, fair, good, or excellent
- Individualized short- and long-term goals
- Written physician acceptance of the specific plan of care

Documentation Required for Daily Notes

Each pulmonary rehabilitation session must be documented and reflect the services provided. Documentation of sessions should include the following:

- Date of service, treatment time, procedure or modality, signature, clinician's credentials
- Notes describing the patient's progress toward treatment goals
- Notes that match billing codes
- Pain scale and location of pain
- Documentation of vital signs during exercise

Other Documentation Needs

In addition to the documentation already mentioned, pulmonary rehabilitation programs should also document the following:

- Rationale for continued need for the unique skill of the rehabilitation services
- Notes from team conferences held at the beginning and at the end of a patient's participation in the program

- Recommendations for a home program plan for collaborative self-management
- Discharge summary and communication to the referring health care provider, which may include the progress made during pulmonary rehabilitation, recommendations for self-care maintenance, symptom management techniques, and a home exercise program
- Postprogram evaluation
- Documentation of continuing physician involvement and direction during the course of the program

The pulmonary rehabilitation medical record must include all necessary documentation. Specific forms should adhere to the requirements of the medical records department in the program's parent institution, even though the format for charting may vary.

Conferences

The effectiveness of the interdisciplinary team depends on an adequate system of communication. The team conference provides the opportunity for this interaction to occur. Team conferences should be held at the beginning and at the end of treatment sessions. The purpose of the conference is for the team to present and discuss the following information:

- History and physical examination data
- Medical test results
- Team members' assessment
- Patient goals
- Specific target or problem areas identified
- Individualized treatment plan
- Patient progress
- Revision of treatment plan if necessary
- Postprogram needs and outcomes

The interdisciplinary team concept provides the patient with the highest quality care possible through the expertise of several disciplines involved and also enhances program quality. Team conference information is necessary to document the patient's progress toward his or her established goals and outcomes. This documentation, which is included in the medical records, must be signed by the medical director, the referring physician, or the program coordinator, as determined by the program's policies and procedures.

Reimbursement

At the time of this writing, pulmonary rehabilitation services are reimbursed by Medicare and Medicaid as incident to physician services. Billing and documentation requirements for all third-party payers must be followed carefully to ensure appropriate reimbursement. Program coordinators, the medical director, and other members of the team should be familiar with current reimbursement guidelines of the Centers for Medicare and Medicaid Services (CMS), Fiscal Intermediaries/Carriers, and other third-party payers. Differences exist throughout the United States in how reimbursement guidelines are applied by various intermediaries and third-party payers. Some services may not be covered, such as nonindividualized education or training, maintenance care, documentation time, duplication of clinical services, films or videos, and treatment that lacks documented medical necessity.

The program coordinator must be familiar with the process of obtaining prior authorization for the pulmonary rehabilitation program by the insurance companies because coverage varies depending on the patient's policy. The coordinator must also become involved with the managed care contracting department to ensure that pulmonary rehabilitation is included during negotiations. Networking with other program coordinators is critical in providing the awareness, knowledge, and support needed to obtain appropriate reimbursement. A close liaison between the coordinator and the facility's business office is necessary to ensure that billing information is complete and accurate. Reimbursement problems that occur must be addressed promptly and effectively.

Strategies for Program Success

Program success depends in part on physician and consumer awareness, which is accomplished through organized strategies. An optimal strategy should address both referring physicians and patients. Strategies that may improve the success of the program include the following:

- Identifying the need for services in the area (competition in the community)
- Tailoring services to patient and community demographics (e.g., setting up a posttransplantation program in a tertiary care center)

- Assessing the opportunities and challenges of the infrastructure (e.g., parking, accessibility)
- Defining and pricing the rehabilitation services
- Identifying a physician referral base
- Promoting the program (e.g., feedback to physicians, patient testimonials)
- Using direct advertising (newspaper, television and radio interviews, wellness fairs, Web sites)
- Using the AACVPR media kit and observing National Pulmonary Rehabilitation Week

The ultimate success of pulmonary rehabilitation services depends on satisfied patients and enthusiastic interdisciplinary team members. Pulmonary rehabilitation must be viewed and marketed from a global perspective, remembering that prevention is integrated into every component of the program.

Postrehabilitation Maintenance Programs

An important goal of pulmonary rehabilitation is to promote long-term maintenance of gains made during the formal pulmonary rehabilitation program, including increased exercise performance. Because exercise performance falls off relatively quickly following resumption of a more sedentary lifestyle, facilitation of long-term exercise training should be a priority. This can be in the form of establishing an exercise maintenance program for graduates of pulmonary rehabilitation. This is often a natural development, given the expertise and dedication of the staff and the availability of space and exercise equipment. Although these are often revenue-negative endeavors, the gains from patient satisfaction and goodwill usually outweigh the relatively minor costs of maintaining the program. Existing exercise maintenance programs might also be appropriate formats for encouraging patients recovering from minor exacerbations of respiratory disease to resume exercise therapy. Patients with less severe functional impairment or comorbidity would be candidates for joining a community gymnasium or exercise program. Structured patient support groups, such as better

breathing clubs, are also useful adjuncts to postrehabilitation, but they do not substitute for exercise maintenance programs.

Continuous Quality Improvement

The goal of continuous quality improvement (CQI) is to enhance patient outcomes. CQI for facility-based programs is frequently directed by the CQI department of the parent facility. A complete description of the CQI process is beyond the scope of these guidelines. However, outcome assessment—which is a necessary component of pulmonary rehabilitation—has a prominent role in helping staff evaluate the overall effectiveness of the program and its components. This can provide valuable feedback information to the staff and promote improvement in the quality of care. Important outcomes and the rationale for their measurement are discussed in chapter 6.

Conclusion

Successful pulmonary rehabilitation, which is reflected in satisfied patients with positive outcomes in several areas, results from a combination of the following factors:

- Effective management techniques and program structure
- A supportive and actively participating medical director
- A motivated and inspiring program coordinator with good leadership and team-building skills
- A dedicated, knowledgeable, and enthusiastic interdisciplinary team
- Accurate and thorough documentation

All of the essential components of pulmonary rehabilitation are only as successful as the people who put them into operation. Success follows the dedicated work of a team of specialized professionals who come together with a common goal of enhancing the lives of the unique and challenging group of patients with chronic pulmonary disease.

Forms, Questionnaires, and Assessments

Initial Interview Form

Name: _____ Date: _____

Address: _____ Phone: _____

Emergency contact: _____ Phone: _____

Age: _____ Sex: _____ Occupation: _____

Height: _____ Weight: _____ Highest level of education: _____

Marital status: _____ Advance directives: _____

Diagnosis: _____ Insurance provider: _____

Referring physician: _____

Primary care physician: _____

Referral source: _____

Chief complaint: _____

History

How many times have you been hospitalized in the last year as a result of lung problems? _____

How many days were you in the hospital in the last year as a result of lung disease? _____

How many E.R. visits have you had in the past year as a result of breathing difficulty? _____

Last hospital admission: _____ Release: _____

Previous hospitalizations: _____

Have you ever attended a pulmonary rehabilitation program? _____

Have you ever had any chest injuries or surgeries?   Yes   No

   Type _____

Do you have any upcoming surgeries?   Yes   No   _____

Do you have any physical limitations that may affect your ability to exercise (sensory loss, amputation, stroke, surgeries,

   fractures, etc.)? _____

Do you have any other medical problems?

Cardiovascular disease _____

Hypertension _____

Diabetes _____

G-I problems _____

Reflux/hiatal hernia _____

Osteoporosis _____

Sinusitis _____

Vision or hearing problems _____

Other _____

Have you ever had or do you have:

Emphysema	_____	Valley fever	_____
Asthma	_____	Tuberculosis	_____
Bronchitis	_____	Pleurisy	_____
Pneumonia	_____	Lung cancer	_____
Bronchiectasis	_____	Sinus trouble	_____
Blood clot in lung	_____	Other	_____
High pressure in lungs	_____		

A.1   Pulmonary rehabilitation initial interview form.

Reprinted courtesy of the Pulmonary Rehabilitation Program at St. Joseph's Hospital and Medical Center, Phoenix, AZ.

Do you have a family history of respiratory disease? _____

Have you ever used tobacco? _____ What form?   Chew   Smoke _____

Do you chew/smoke now? _____ How long did you use or have you used tobacco? _____

When did you stop chewing/smoking?_____

If you are still smoking, do you plan to quit? _____

Do you live with any smokers?_____

Other substance abuse? _____

Have you ever been exposed to:

Asbestos dust	Yes	No	Paint fumes	Yes	No
Cotton dust	Yes	No	Plastic fumes	Yes	No
Mining dust	Yes	No	Solvent fumes	Yes	No
Other dust	Yes	No	Other fumes	Yes	No

Do you consume alcohol? _____ How much? _____

Do you have any allergies (food, pollen, drugs, etc.)? _____

How many colds do you get per year?_____

Vaccines: Flu   Yes   No   Pneumonia   Yes   No

Do you ever have chest pain? _____ Location _____

   Type of pain _____ Frequency _____

Have you ever had a heart attack?_____ When? _____

Major Symptomatology

What are your symptoms today? _____

What were your symptoms last year?_____

What were your symptoms 5 years ago? _____

When did you realize that you had lung problems?_____

Disease Impact

Do you sleep flat or with your head elevated? _____

   If elevated, how high? _____

Do you awaken during the night? _____ How often? _____

   Why? _____

Do your ankles ever swell up? _____ When?_____

Do you cough?_____ What part of the day?_____

Do you cough up sputum?_____ When? _____

   Describe _____

   Have you ever coughed up blood? _____

MRC Dyspnea Scale

[0] _____ Breathless with strenuous exercise

[1] _____ Shortness of breath when hurrying on the level or walking up a slight hill

[2] _____ Walks slower than people of the same age on the level because of breathlessness, or has to stop for breath when walking at own pace on the level

[3] _____ Stops for breath after walking about 100 yards or after a few minutes on the level

[4] _____ Too breathless to leave the house or when dressing or undressing

(continued)

A.1   *(continued)*

Do you use oxygen?_____ How often?_____ Liters per minute_____

Type of oxygen delivery system _____ Supplier_____

Are you on any home respiratory therapy?_____ Type_____

   How do you clean the equipment? _____

Do you have trouble eating? _____ Why? _____

Do you have trouble gaining or losing weight? _____

Have you experienced a recent weight change?_____

Do you have a special diet?_____

Are you able to care for yourself? _____

Are you able to take care of your home? _____

Do you exercise? _____ If yes, how?_____ How often? _____

Do you have exercise equipment? _____ Type _____

Has your physician limited your activities?_____

Do you have any special interests or hobbies?_____

What activities does your breathing difficulty prevent you from doing that you would like to do? _____

Does your breathing interfere with your ability to have sexual relations? _____

Are others close to you affected by your health?_____

   If yes, how? _____

Are you affected by trying to live up to others' expectations? _____

   How? _____

Do you find yourself worrying daily? _____ occasionally?_____ almost never? _____

Does your income cover your expenses and needs? _____

Do you live alone? _____

Do you have transportation? _____ What form?_____

How do you heat and cool your home? _____

Do you have any pets?_____

Medications

Type	Amount	Frequency
_____	_____	_____
_____	_____	_____
_____	_____	_____
_____	_____	_____
_____	_____	_____
_____	_____	_____
_____	_____	_____
_____	_____	_____
_____	_____	_____
_____	_____	_____
_____	_____	_____

Medication compliance: Yes No

M.D.I. technique: _____

Spacer: Yes No   Type:_____   Needs training: Yes No

A.1 *(continued)*

Observations

Color _____ Skin turgor _____

Mentation _____ Energy level _____

Nutritional status _____

Blood pressure _____ Pulse _____ Edema _____

Respirations (rate, rhythm, depth) _____

Accessory breather? _____ Pursed lips? _____

Abdominal breathing? _____ Other _____

Auscultation _____

Data From Patient's Records

FEV$_1$ _____ FEV$_1$/FVC _____ ABGs _____ Hb/Hct _____

Alb _____ EKG _____ Other _____

Client's Stated Goals

Please state your goals or what you expect to achieve from this rehabilitation program.

_____

_____

Patient's signature _____

Estimated Learning Ability

_____ No baseline, slow learner   _____ Some baseline, slow learner

_____ No baseline, good learner   _____ Some baseline, good learner

_____ Needs only comprehensive review and reinforcement

Degree of motivation _____

Candidacy: Accept _____   Reject _____

Evaluator's signature _____

A.1   *(continued)*

Participant Questionnaire

Date: _____ Physician: _____

Name: _____

Address: _____

City/state: _____ Zip: _____ Phone: _____

Age: _____ Birth date: _____ Marital status: M   S   W   D

Spouse's name: _____

Social Security #: _____ Medicare #: _____

Insurance: _____

_____

Diagnosis: _____

Living Situation _____ House _____ Apartment _____ Mobile home _____ Condo

Level: _____ Single _____ Multi

Entrance: _____ Incline _____ Stair(s) # _____

Household members: _____

(Relationships & names) _____

Household pets: _____

(Types & names) _____

Usual household duties I perform: _____ Cooking _____ Cleaning _____ Finances _____ Laundry

_____ Transportation _____ Yard work _____ Grocery shopping

My major source(s) of support: (names and relationships) _____

Transportation _____ Currently drive _____ Rely on family _____ Rely on friends

_____ Use public transportation _____ Is a real problem for me

Occupational History

Current or former occupation: _____

Retirement/disability date: _____

Occupational exposure: _____ Welding _____ Pottery _____ Asbestos _____ Mines/foundry

_____ Gas/fumes _____ Quarry _____ Sandblasting _____ Chemicals _____ Dust

Educational History

The last grade I completed was: _____

I learn information best by: _____ Explanation _____ Reading _____ Video/TV _____ Computer _____ Demonstration

Medical History

(Please check those that apply; mark with F if family history exists)

_____ Asthma   _____ Tuberculosis   _____ Fractures (specify) _____

_____ Chronic bronchitis   _____ Diabetes   _____ Cancer

_____ Emphysema   _____ Sinus problems   _____ Pneumonia

_____ Bronchiectasis   _____ High blood pressure   _____ Heart disease

_____ Osteoporosis   _____ Arthritis   _____ Sarcoidosis

_____ Cystic fibrosis   _____ Pulmonary fibrosis   _____ Collapsed lung

A.2 Pulmonary rehabilitation participant questionnaire.

Adapted from Pulmonary Rehabilitation Programs at Long Beach Memorial Medical Center, Long Beach, CA, Mt. Diablo Medical Center, Concord, CA, and Union Hospital, Dover, OH.

Allergy History

I have seen an allergist. ـــــ Yes ـــــ No

Was skin testing performed? ـــــ Yes ـــــ No

I am allergic to the following:

Food(s): _____

Medications: _____

Environmental: ـــــ Dust ـــــ Mold ـــــ Pollens ـــــ Grass Other: _____

I have difficulty when exposed to the following environmental irritants:

ـــــ Dust ـــــ Smog ـــــ Solvents ـــــ Humidity ـــــ Perfumes/colognes

ـــــ Rapid changes in temperature ـــــ Tobacco smoke ـــــ Wind ـــــ Other: _____

Vaccine History

I receive the flu vaccine annually. ـــــ Yes ـــــ No

If no, why not? _____

I have received the pneumonia vaccine. ـــــ Yes ـــــ No

Year received: _____

Smoking History

ـــــ I have never smoked.

ـــــ I have smoked in the past but do not smoke now.

Year started: _____ Year quit: _____

Number of packs smoked per day: _____

ـــــ I am currently a smoker.

Number of packs smoked per day: _____

Exposure to secondhand smoke: ـــــ None ـــــ Home ـــــ Work ـــــ Social situations

Pulmonary Health History

Cough: ـــــ Yes ـــــ No

ـــــ A.M. ـــــ P.M. ـــــ Nighttime ـــــ Around the clock

Mucus: Normal color: _____ ـــــ Thick ـــــ Thin ـــــ Moderate

Amount/day: ___ 1 tsp. ___ 1-2 tsp. ___ 1 Tbsp. ___ 1/4 cup ___ 1/2 cup ___ 1 cup ___ >1 cup

When: ___ A.M. ___ P.M. ___ Around the clock

I use the following to help me raise my mucus:

ـــــ Drink warm liquids   ـــــ Inhalers

ـــــ Aerosol treatments   ـــــ Chest percussion

ـــــ Postural drainage   ـــــ Increase my fluids

I have coughed up blood. ـــــ Yes ـــــ No When: _____

I have taken steroid pills (e.g., prednisone). ـــــ Yes ـــــ No

Length of time: _____ Last date: _____ Highest dose: _____

I experience the following:

ـــــ Chest pain   ـــــ Dizziness/unsteadiness   ـــــ Hoarseness

ـــــ Fatigue   ـــــ Ankle swelling   ـــــ Weight change

ـــــ Wheezing

Known trigger factors: _____

(continued)

A.2 *(continued)*

I have been on a ventilator (respirator) in an intensive care unit. _____ Yes _____ No   Last date: _____

What I remember most about that experience is: _____

_____

I see my lung doctor every (please give a time frame): _____

Pulmonary Infections

Number/year: _____

Antibiotic usually taken: _____

I know I have an infection when: _____

Pulmonary Hospitalizations

Number in past year: _____   Number in previous year: _____

Emergency Room Visits for Pulmonary Reasons

Number in past year: _____   Number in previous year: _____

Shortness of Breath

I have experienced shortness of breath since: _____

My breathing is most difficult: _____ Early A.M.   _____ A.M.   _____ P.M.   _____ Bedtime

I do the following to decrease or avoid being short of breath:

_____ Stop and rest	_____ Use aerosol machine
_____ Use inhalers	_____ Use belly or diaphragm breathing
_____ Use a fan or air conditioner	_____ Open windows
_____ Remove myself from the irritant	_____ Limit my activity
_____ Practice a relaxation technique	_____ Avoid exposure to irritants
_____ Check the air pollution forecast	_____ Check my peak flow
_____ Use pursed-lip breathing	_____ Avoid tobacco smoke exposure

Dietary History

Current height: _____   Current weight: _____

I have recently had a change in my weight. _____ Yes _____ No

Gained _____ pounds   Lost _____ pounds

Over this period of time: _____

I can attribute this weight change to: _____

I would like to weigh: _____ pounds

I follow the following type of diet:

_____ No special diet	_____ Low saturated fat	_____ Ulcer
_____ Low sodium (salt)	_____ Caloric restriction	_____ Hiatal hernia
_____ Low cholesterol	_____ Diabetic	_____ Other _____

My appetite is: _____ Good _____ Fair _____ Poor

I drink this amount of each of these a day:

Water _____	Sodas _____	Coffee _____
Tea _____	Wine _____	Hard liquor _____
Milk _____	Juice _____	Beer _____

A.2 *(continued)*

I have difficulty with: chewing   ____ Yes   ____ No

                        swallowing ____ Yes   ____ No

                        digestion   ____ Yes   ____ No

I take vitamins.   ____ Yes ____ No

    If yes, please list: _____

Sleeping History

Usual bedtime _____ Usual time of waking up _____

Naps taken during the day: Number: _____ Length: _____

Number of pillows used when sleeping: _____

Medications/strategies used to help me sleep: _____

Medication name/strength	Amount and frequency on a daily basis	Time(s) of the day medication taken	Purpose of medication	Comments that you have
Example: 1. Albuterol	2 puffs 4 times a day	6 A.M., 2 P.M., 6 P.M., 11 P.M.	improve breathing	works well
Example: 2. Lasix 40 mg	1 tablet once a day	in the morning usually 6 A.M.	blood pressure	

Activities of Daily Living

Use this shortness of breath scale to answer the following questions:

Scale: 0 = None; 1 = Minimal; 2 = Moderate; 3 = Great; 4 = Unable

To what degree do you get short of breath at rest? ____

To what degree do you get short of breath when climbing stairs? ____

How many stairs? ____

To what degree do you get short of breath during the following activities:

____ Eating

____ Simple personal care (washing face, combing hair, etc.)

____ Taking full bath or shower

____ Dressing

____ Picking up or straightening up

____ Sweeping or vacuuming

____ Shopping

____ Laundry

____ Cooking and doing dishes

____ Walking around your house

____ Walking your own pace on level surface

____ Walking one block

____ Walking with others your age

____ Walking up a slight hill

(continued)

A.2 *(continued)*

Activity/Exercise History

____ Yes ____ No   I currently do purposeful walking ____ days a week for ____ minutes.

____ Yes ____ No   I do calisthenics ____ days/week.

____ Yes ____ No   I do purposeful exercise programs.

The following things limit my ability to remain active:

____ Shortness of breath   ____ Lightheadedness

____ Fatigue   ____ Joint problems (specify): _____

I have the following exercise equipment available:

____ None

____ Stationary bike   ____ Treadmill   ____ Stair stepper

____ Pool   ____ Weights   ____ Other: _____

Equipment/Assistive Device History

I use the following items:

____ Walker   ____ Eyeglasses

____ Wheelchair   ____ Electric cart

____ Cane   ____ Hearing aid

____ Four-point quad cane   ____ Other: _____

Respiratory Home Care Equipment History

I use the following items: Frequency used:

____ Peak flow meter   _____

____ Aerosol machine (e.g., Pulmoaide)   _____

____ Suction machine   _____

____ Ventilator   _____

____ Mechanical chest percussor   _____

____ PEP valve   _____

____ Oxygen: ____Flow rate   System: ____ Concentrator

                                     ____ Tank

                                     ____ Liquid

                                     ____ Pulse

Oxygen used: ____ Continuously   ____ Only when I need it   ____ With sleep only   ____ With exercise only

            ____ With sleep and exercise

I change my oxygen tubing every:

____ Week   ____ 2 weeks   ____ 3-4 weeks   ____ 1-2 months   ____ Oops! I didn't know I needed to change it.

My home care equipment vendor is: _____

Day-to-Day Living

I am sexually active   ____ Yes   ____ No

My present interests and hobbies are: _____

Former interests and hobbies in which I can no longer participate are: _____

This is what I do for fun: _____

I would describe my present temperament (mood) as: _____
(examples: worried, sad, impatient, frustrated, depressed, anxious, contented, cheerful, etc.)

A.2 (continued)

116

This is what makes me feel this way: _____

I use the following to relax:

_____ Read	_____ Alcohol	_____ Other: _____
_____ Deep breathing	_____ Yoga	
_____ Smoke	_____ Pursed-lip breathing	
_____ TV	_____ Tranquilizer	

This has been the most difficult adjustment for me because of my lung disease:

_____

This is how my lung disease has affected how I feel about myself:

_____

My goals for completing pulmonary rehabilitation are: _____

_____

A.2 *(continued)*

Outpatient Pulmonary Rehabilitation Program

Physician Referral Form

Name: _____ DOB: _____

Diagnosis: _____

1. I agree to have my patient participate in the _____ Outpatient Pulmonary Rehabilitation Program.

2. I am aware that certain diagnostic data (such as PFTs, 6-minute walk test, CXR, EKG, cardiopulmonary exercise test) may be required and will be requested by the program director if not already available.

3. I agree to have my patient counseled in all areas related to pulmonary rehabilitation.

4. I agree to continue the regular care of my patient throughout his/her participation in the program.

Physician signature: _____

Phone: _____ Special considerations:

Fax: _____ _____

Date: _____ _____

_____

A.3 Outpatient pulmonary rehabilitation physician referral form.

Used by permission from St. Francis Hospital and Medical Center, Hartford, CT.

**Pulmonary Rehabilitation
Physical Therapy Evaluation**

Patient name: _____

MRN: _____

MD: _____

Today's date: _____ Time in: _____ Time out: _____ Age: _____ ❑ F ❑ M

Diagnosis: _____ Onset: _____

_____ Onset: _____

_____ Onset: _____

PMH: ❑ Hypertension ❑ Diabetes ❑ Cancer ❑ Osteoporosis ❑ Cardiac ❑ Fracture ❑ Surgery

❑ H/O falls ❑ Signs of abuse/neglect

Other: _____

_____

Current medications: _____

_____

❑ Bone density test: _____ Exercise test complete: ❑ Yes, max watts: _____ ❑ No, scheduled: _____

Pulmonary rehabilitation history: _____

_____

Home exercise: _____

Mental status: _____

Social/Family status: _____

Three greatest difficulties: _____ , _____ , _____

Patient goals: _____ , _____ , _____

Cough: _____

Oxygen use: *At rest:* _____ by _____ *Exercise:* _____ by _____ *Sleep:* _____ by _____

Smoking history: _____

Pain

Location: _____ Duration: _____ Character: _____

Current: _____/10 Best: _____/10 Worst: _____/10 Increases with: _____ Decreases with: _____

Edema: ❑ No ❑ Yes Location: _____ Exacerbated by: _____

Examination

Auscultation: _____

Breathing pattern: ❑ Diaphragmatic: _____ ❑ Accessory muscle use: _____ ❑ Pursed Lips: _____

Range of motion: UE: _____ LE: _____

Strength: UE: _____ LE: _____

Posture/Skin/Physical Characteristics/Other: _____

Gait: _____

Foot evaluation: ❑ Overpronator ❑ Normal pronator ❑ Supinator Given shoe list: ❑ Yes ❑ No

Other: _____

A.4 Pulmonary rehabilitation physical therapy evaluation form.

Used by permission from Duke University Hospital.

Patient name: _____ MRN: _____

Precautions

❑ Aspiration
❑ Incisional
❑ Osteoporosis
❑ Hypertension
❑ Hernia
❑ Musculoskeletal
❑ Cardiac
❑ Diabetes
❑ Risk of falls
❑ Other:_____

Problems

❑ Retained secretions
❑ Ineffective breathing pattern
❑ Limited range of motion
❑ Postural deviations
❑ Decrease mobility
❑ Pain
❑ Oxygen desaturation
❑ Decreased strength
❑ Altered mental status
❑ Altered nutritional status
❑ Smoking
❑ Decreased functional level (ADLs, self care)
❑ Other:_____

Treatment/Plan

❑ Cough techniques
❑ Flutter/Acapella/Vest
❑ PD and percussion
❑ 3-day trial pulmonary hygiene
❑ Breathing retraining
❑ Postural exercises
❑ Chair exercises
❑ Ice
❑ Hot packs
❑ TENS
❑ Nutritional consult
❑ Smoking cessation consult
❑ General conditioning
❑ Progressive ambulation
❑ Strengthening
❑ Stretching
❑ Home exercise program
❑ Footwear education
❑ Referral to outpatient physical therapy

Special Considerations

❑ Use pillows/wedge for floor exercise
❑ Incisional precautions until _____
❑ No upper body flexion or rotation
❑ Give osteoporosis handout
❑ BP daily
❑ Monitor blood glucose
❑ Preexercise   ❑ Postexercise
❑ Other: _____

Goals Developed Collaboratively With Patient:

Short-Term Goal: In _____ *weeks patient will:*

1. Ambulate _____ feet in 6 min. with _____ rests and _____ assist with _____ assistive device
2. _____
3. _____
4. _____

Long-Term Goal: In _____ *weeks patient will:*

1. Ambulate _____ feet in _____ min. with _____ rests and _____ assist with _____ assistive device
2. _____
3. _____
4. _____

Patient's rehab potential: ❑ Poor   ❑ Fair   ❑ Good   ❑ Excellent

Frequency of treatment: _____   Duration of program: _____

Physical therapist: _____   Date: _____

Physician's Medicare Certification: I certify that this patient is under my care. The above treatment plan of care has been reviewed by me and I authorize it to be implemented for the next 30 days.

Physician's signature: _____   Date: _____

A.4 *(continued)*

1.5–2 METs

Walking 1 mph

Standing

Driving automobile

Sitting at desk or typing

2–3 METs

Walking 2.5–3 mph

Dusting furniture, light housework

Preparing a meal

3–4 METs

Sweeping

Vacuuming

Ironing

Walking 3 mph

Golfing (power cart)

Pushing light lawnmower

4–5 METs

Calisthenics

Cycling outdoors 6 mph

Painting

Golfing (carrying clubs)

Playing tennis (doubles)

5–6 METs

Walking 4 mph

Digging in garden

Ice or roller skating 9 mph

Doing carpentry

6–7 METs

Stationary cycling (vigorous)

Playing tennis (singles)

Shoveling snow

Mowing lawn (nonpowered)

A.5 Representative levels of energy expenditure (in METs).

Note: One MET is the level of energy expenditure at rest, or approximately 3.5 ml/kg/min of oxygen consumption.

Nutritional Assessment

Name: _____ Date: _____

Height: _____ Weight: _____

What is your "usual" adult weight? _____

Have you gained or lost any weight recently?   No   Yes   How much? _____

Over what period of time? _____

What do you attribute it to? _____

Have you noticed any changes in your eating habits since your pulmonary problems began? _____

If so, describe them: _____

Do you follow any of these dietary restrictions?

    Low salt   Diabetic   Gout   Ulcer   Low fat/cholesterol   Hiatal hernia   Other:_____

Caloric intake: _____

How would you describe your appetite?_____

Is this usual for you?   No   Yes

Do you take vitamin or mineral supplements?   No   Yes   Specify name, strength, and frequency.

_____

_____

Do you have any food allergies?   No   Yes   What are they?

_____

_____

Describe any problems you have with:

  Dental: _____

  Chewing: _____

  Swallowing:_____

  Digestion: _____

  Constipation or diarrhea: _____

  Bloating: _____

  Nausea: _____

  Fatigue: _____

  Shortness of breath: _____

How many ounces of the following fluids do you drink:

	Daily	Weekly	Rarely
Water	_____	_____	_____
Soft drinks*	_____	_____	_____
Juice	_____	_____	_____
Milk	_____	_____	_____
Coffee*	_____	_____	_____
Tea*	_____	_____	_____
Beer	_____	_____	_____
Wine	_____	_____	_____
Hard liquor	_____	_____	_____

*Caffeine/decaffeinated

(continued)

A.6 Nutritional assessment form.

Reprinted courtesy of the Pulmonary Rehabilitation Program at Mt. Diablo Medical Center, Concord, CA.

FOR STAFF USE ONLY:

%IBW: _____   BMI: _____

Weight change: Mild   Moderate   Severe

Supplements?_____

Available labs: Albumin _____   Cholesterol _____   Other _____

Possible drug or nutrient interactions?

_____

_____

Comments:

_____

_____

Assessment and recommendations:

_____

_____

_____

_____

Date: _____   Dietitian: _____, RD

A.6 *(continued)*

Reprinted courtesy of the Pulmonary Rehabilitation Program at Mt. Diablo Medical Center, Concord, CA.

	True	False	Not Sure
1. The diaphragm is a muscle that does most of the work of breathing.	1	2	3
2. Emphysema is a disease that primarily affects air sacs (alveoli).	1	2	3
3. "Pursed-lip breathing" helps prevent small airways from collapsing.	1	2	3
4. People with chronic lung disease can abruptly stop taking a steroid medication such as prednisone at any time without ill effects.	1	2	3
5. Changing the flow rate on oxygen equipment can be dangerous for a person with chronic lung disease.	1	2	3
6. For a person with chronic lung disease, eating six small meals a day rather than three large meals can help to reduce shortness of breath during and after meals.	1	2	3
7. For a person with chronic lung disease, foods that are high in protein, such as fish, are an important part of the diet.	1	2	3
8. Drinking water has no effect on the mucus in the lungs.	1	2	3
9. A person with chronic lung disease should rinse out the mouth after using a steroid metered-dose inhaler.	1	2	3
10. When climbing stairs, a person with chronic lung disease should hold his or her breath briefly while taking a step.	1	2	3
11. For people with chronic lung disease, the most efficient method of completing a task is to work quickly in short bursts and to take frequent rests.	1	2	3
12. During activity, people with chronic lung disease should exhale when they exert themselves.	1	2	3
13. If someone with chronic lung disease is taking antibiotics, it is fine for that person to stop taking them when he or she feels better.	1	2	3
14. During diaphragmatic breathing, it is important for a person with chronic lung disease to pull in the abdomen during inhalation.	1	2	3
15. It is important for a person with chronic lung disease to keep the shoulder muscles relaxed to decrease the amount of oxygen used for breathing.	1	2	3
16. A bronchodilator, such as Albuterol, gets rid of infection.	1	2	3

A.7   Sample quiz for patients with chronic lung disease.

Adapted by permission from Y. Scherer, L. Schmeider, and S. Shimmell. 1995. "Outpatient instruction for individuals with COPD," *Perspectives in Respiratory Nursing* 6 (3):3.

Pulmonary Rehabilitation Perioperative Education Sessions and Support Group

Name: _____

Patient ID#: _____

Education Sessions

Date

_____ Spacers/MDIs

_____ Pulmonary issues

_____ ABG/PFTs

_____ Nutrition

_____ Home equipment

_____ Exercise responses

_____ Urinary incontinence

_____ Medications

_____ Charting/Inhalers

_____ Lung disease pathology

_____ Anatomy and physiology I

_____ Anatomy and physiology II

_____ Preoperative aspects (pre only)

_____ Transplant medications (post)

_____ Transplant issues (1st Monday of each month, 11:30 A.M.)

_____ Transplant medications (pre-op participants only, 3rd Monday of each month, 11:30 A.M.)

Date

_____ Oxygen

_____ Chest PT

_____ Carolina Organ Procurement Association

_____ Doctor's day

_____ Osteoporosis

_____ Graduate program

_____ Home program

_____ Graduation

_____ Travel issues

_____ Topic of choice

_____ Progress review

_____ _____

_____ _____

_____ _____

Support Group
(List dates)

_____ _____ _____ _____

_____ _____ _____ _____

Monday/Wednesday lectures: 3:45-4:30

Tuesday support group: Intensive 2:45-3:30

Perioperative 3:45-4:30

Thursday lectures: 2:45-3:30

Friday lectures: 2:15

All lectures will be held in the Meltzer room of the fitness building.

*If it has been three months since you last heard a lecture, it may need to be repeated.

A.8 Pulmonary rehabilitation perioperative education sessions and support group.

appendix b

Measures for Promoting Maintenance

Follow-up care, or maintenance, provides the opportunity for pulmonary rehabilitation participants to maintain or even continue improving their symptom management, functional status, and quality of life. After participants' graduation from the structured, supervised pulmonary rehabilitation program, a process for the maintenance of knowledge, skills, and enhanced performance is needed. With the assistance of the rehabilitation staff, patients can locate services that will meet their maintenance needs.

Many programs offer postrehabilitation maintenance. Alternatively, similar programs can often be found in most communities. For those rehabilitation facilities offering maintenance programs, many patients will return regularly because of principles taught during the formal process and perhaps because of the bonding that usually occurs between the patient and the staff. Patients receive long-term support when they return to the facility.

However, for various reasons some rehabilitation facilities may not be able to offer structured postrehabilitation maintenance. Additionally, the patient may not be able to return regularly because of distance or cost. In this case, the rehabilitation staff could assist the patient in locating a facility (preferably in the patient's community) for exercise maintenance.

Regardless of whether a patient attends a structured postrehabilitation maintenance program, program staff should provide a written individualized home exercise plan prior to the patient's completion

of the program. This written plan should include the following:

- Self-monitoring guidelines for target heart rate and appropriate dyspnea levels during exercise
- Current level of exercise and exercise goals
- Exercise log, with specific instructions for its completion
- Reminders to follow medication instructions, nutrition recommendations, breathing techniques, and other home recommendations

Continued physical and functional gains are the goals of maintenance. These goals cannot be achieved if exercise is discontinued. The saying "variety is the spice of life" is not just a cliché but a useful guideline for keeping participants interested and motivated to exercise on a consistent basis. An enthusiastic, creative, and supportive rehabilitation staff is critical in getting pulmonary rehabilitation participants to continue in a maintenance exercise program. Appealing and innovative options for maintenance exercise include the following:

- Treadmills or stationary bicycles
- Upper body ergometry and circuit weight training
- Elastic bands
- Modified low-impact aerobic exercise routines or dance steps

- Group game activities
- Pool exercises
- Walking
- Climbing stairs

Another incentive for maintaining and increasing an exercise capacity is to participate in local Olympic-style competition, sponsored regionally by the affiliate societies of the American Association of Cardiovascular and Pulmonary Rehabilitation (AACVPR). These games are held as often as yearly in some regions. Every three years, AACVPR sponsors the International Heart and Lung Games, which include teams from across the country. These activities encourage lung patients of all ages to undergo physical training before participating in these events. Other options for the graduates may be enrollment in fitness clubs, YMCAs, and senior centers. For all of the previous options, an individualized, goal-oriented physical activity program is extremely valuable in improving compliance and continuing physical and functional gains.

Psychosocial maintenance and follow-up should not be overlooked. Following are some examples:

- Support groups for participants and significant others
- Well spouses' support groups
- Better Breathers' Club of the American Lung Association
- Social outings (e.g., bus trips, parties, picnics, movies, cruises)
- Newsletters
- Cards (e.g., birthday, get well)
- Volunteer work in the pulmonary rehabilitation program

Involvement in activities designed to assist others helps the patient to hold onto relationships that facilitate communication and fellowship, increase self-esteem, and promote a positive attitude.

The use of home care services is an option for pulmonary participants when needed, but it depends on insurance coverage. Home care services allow medical services to be rendered in the comfort and convenience of the patient's home. Following are some examples:

- Evaluation of the participant's need for adaptive equipment and medical supplies
- Home ventilator management
- IV therapy
- Wound care
- Respiratory equipment evaluation, use instruction, and cleaning
- Psychosocial support
- Monitoring of the pulmonary rehabilitation home recommendations

The need for home care has been well established and continues to grow. With the increasing emphasis on providing care in a less costly setting, the rehabilitation team can be an essential part of the overall reduction in health care expenditures by keeping abreast of the community services available to their participants.

A postprogram follow-up questionnaire may be used to gather information on how the participant is complying with the home program. The information gathered may be tabulated and used for continuous quality improvement.

If the rehabilitation staff continues to see the patient during maintenance, opportunities are provided for ongoing interaction between the participant's primary care physician and the program. If follow-up evaluations are performed by the rehabilitation facility, reports can be sent to the referring or primary care physician regarding the patient's progress and compliance with the home exercise program, in addition to information gathered from the follow-up evaluation and questionnaires. This process helps to ensure a continued excellent relationship between patients' primary care physicians and pulmonary rehabilitation programs, while also improving patients' compliance.

American Thoracic Society Statement: Guidelines for the Six-Minute Walk Test

This official statement of the American Thoracic Society was approved by the ATS Board of Directors in March 2002.

Contents

Purpose and Scope

This statement provides practical guidelines for the 6-minute walk test (6MWT). Specifically, it reviews indications, details factors that influence results, presents a brief step-by-step protocol, outlines safety measures, describes proper patient preparation and procedures, and offers guidelines for clinical interpretation of results. These recommendations are not intended to limit the use of alternative protocols for research studies. We do not discuss the general topic of clinical exercise testing.

As with other American Thoracic Society statements on pulmonary function testing, these guidelines come out of a consensus conference. Drafts were prepared by two members (P.L.E. and R.J.Z.) and were based on a comprehensive Medline literature search from 1970 through 2001, augmented by suggestions from other committee members. Each draft responded to comments from the working committee. The guidelines follow previously published methods as closely as possible and provide a rationale for each specific recommendation. The final recommendations represent a consensus of the committee. The committee recommends that these guidelines be reviewed in five years and in the meantime encourages further research in areas of controversy.

Background

There are several modalities available for the objective evaluation of functional exercise capacity. Some provide a very complete assessment of all systems involved in exercise performance (high tech), whereas others provide basic information but are low tech and are simpler to perform. The modality used should be chosen based on the clinical question to be addressed and on available resources. The most popular clinical exercise tests in order of increasing complexity are stair climbing, a 6MWT, a shuttle-walk test, detection of exercise-induced asthma, a cardiac stress test (e.g., Bruce protocol), and a cardiopulmonary exercise test.[1,2] Other professional organizations have published standards for cardiac stress testing.[3,4]

Assessment of functional capacity has traditionally been done by merely asking patients the following: "How many flights of stairs can you climb or how many blocks can you walk?" However, patients vary in their recollection and may report overestimations or underestimations of their true functional capacity. Objective measurements are usually better than self-reports. In the early 1960s, Balke developed a simple test to evaluate the functional capacity by measuring the distance walked during a defined period of time.[5] A 12-minute field performance test was then developed to evaluate the level of physical fitness of healthy individuals.[6] The walking test was also adapted to assess disability in patients with chronic bronchitis.[7] In an attempt to accommodate patients with respiratory disease for whom walking 12 minutes was too exhausting, a 6-minute walk was found to perform as well as the 12-minute walk.[8] A recent review of functional walking tests concluded that "the 6MWT is easy to administer, better tolerated, and more reflective of activities of daily living than the other walk tests."[9]

The 6MWT is a practical simple test that requires a 100-ft hallway but no exercise equipment or advanced training for technicians. Walking is an activity performed daily by all but the most severely impaired patients. This test measures the distance that a patient can quickly walk on a flat, hard surface in a period of 6 minutes (the 6MWD). It evaluates the global and integrated responses of all the systems involved during exercise, including the pulmonary and cardiovascular systems, systemic circulation, peripheral circulation, blood, neuromuscular units, and muscle metabolism. It does not provide specific information on the function of each of the different organs and systems involved in exercise or the mechanism of exercise limitation, as is possible with maximal cardiopulmonary exercise testing. The self-paced 6MWT assesses the submaximal level of functional capacity. Most patients do not achieve maximal exercise capacity during the 6MWT; instead, they choose their own intensity of exercise and are allowed to stop and rest during the test. However, because most activities of daily living are performed at submaximal levels of exertion, the 6MWD may better reflect the functional exercise level for daily physical activities.

Indications and Limitations

The strongest indication for the 6MWT is for measuring the response to medical interventions in patients with moderate to severe heart or lung disease. The 6MWT has also been used as a one-time measure of functional status of patients, as well as a predictor of morbidity and mortality (see table 1 for a list of these indications). The fact that investigators have used the 6MWT in these settings does not prove that the test is clinically useful (or the best test) for determining functional capacity or changes in functional capacity due to an intervention in patients with these diseases. Further studies are necessary to determine the utility of the 6MWT in various clinical situations.

Formal cardiopulmonary exercise testing provides a global assessment of the exercise response, an objective determination of functional capacity and impairment, determination of the appropriate intensity needed to perform prolonged exercise, quantification of factors limiting exercise, and a definition of the underlying pathophysiologic mechanisms such as the contribution of different organ systems involved in exercise. The 6MWT does not determine peak oxygen uptake, diagnose the cause of dyspnea on exertion, or evaluate the causes or mechanisms of exercise limitation.[1,2] The information provided by a 6MWT should be considered complementary to cardiopulmonary exercise testing, not a replacement for it. Despite the difference between these two functional tests, some good correlations between them have been reported. For

Table 1   Indications for the Six-Minute Walk Test

Pretreatment and Posttreatment Comparisons
Lung transplantation[9,10]
Lung resection[11]
Lung volume reduction surgery[12,13]
Pulmonary rehabilitation[14,15]
COPD[16-18]
Pulmonary hypertension
Heart failure[19,20]

Functional Status (Single Measurement)
COPD[21,22]
Cystic fibrosis[23,24]
Heart failure[25-27]
Peripheral vascular disease[28,29]
Fibromyalgia[30]
Older patients[31]

Predictor of Morbidity and Mortality
Heart failure[32,33]
COPD[34,35]
Primary pulmonary hypertension[10,36]

Definition of abbreviation: COPD = chronic obstructive pulmonary disease.

example, a significant correlation ($r = 0.73$) between 6MWD and peak oxygen uptake has been reported for patients with end-stage lung diseases.[36,37]

In some clinical situations, the 6MWT provides information that may be a better index of the patient's ability to perform daily activities than is peak oxygen uptake; for example, 6MWD correlates better with formal measures of quality of life.[38] Changes in 6MWD after therapeutic interventions correlate with subjective improvement in dyspnea.[39,40] The reproducibility of the 6MWD (with a coefficient of variation of approximately 8%) appears to be better than the reproducibility of 1-second forced expiratory volume in patients with chronic obstructive pulmonary disease (COPD).[8,41-43] Questionnaire indices of functional status have a larger short-term variability (22-33%) than does the 6MWD.[37]

The shuttle-walking test is similar to the 6MWT, but it uses an audio signal from a tape cassette to direct the walking pace of the patient back and forth on a 100-m course.[44-47] The walking speed is increased every minute, and the test ends when the patient cannot reach the turnaround point within the required time. The exercise performed is similar to a symptom-limited, maximal, incremental treadmill test. An advantage of the shuttle walking test is that it has a better correlation with peak oxygen uptake than the 6MWD. Disadvantages include less validation, less widespread use, and more potential for cardiovascular problems.

Contraindications

Absolute contraindications for the 6MWT include the following: unstable angina during the previous month and myocardial infarction during the previous month. Relative contraindications include a resting heart rate of more than 120, a systolic blood pressure of more than 180 mmHg, and a diastolic blood pressure of more than 100 mmHg.

Patients with any of these findings should be referred to the physician ordering or supervising the test for individual clinical assessment and a decision about the conduct of the test. The results from a resting electrocardiogram done during the previous 6 months should also be reviewed before testing. Stable exertional angina is not an absolute contraindication for a 6MWT, but patients with these symptoms should perform the test after using their antiangina medication, and rescue nitrate medication should be readily available.

Rationale

Patients with the previously mentioned risk factors may be at increased risk for arrhythmias or cardiovascular collapse during testing. However, each patient determines the intensity of their exercise, and the test (without electrocardiogram monitoring) has been performed in thousands of older persons[31,48-50] and thousands of patients with heart failure or cardiomyopathy[32,51,52] without serious adverse events. The contraindications listed previously here were used by study investigators based on their impressions of the general safety of the 6MWT and their desire to be prudent, but it is unknown whether adverse events would occur if such patients performed a 6MWT; they are, therefore, listed as relative contraindications.

Safety Issues

1. Testing should be performed in a location where a rapid, appropriate response to an emergency is possible. The appropriate location of a crash cart should be determined by the physician supervising the facility.
2. Supplies that must be available include oxygen, sublingual nitroglycerine, aspirin, and albuterol (metered dose inhaler or nebulizer).

A telephone or other means should be in place to enable a call for help.

3. The technician should be certified in cardiopulmonary resuscitation with a minimum of Basic Life Support by an American Health Association–approved cardiopulmonary resuscitation course. Advanced cardiac life support certification is desirable. Training, experience, and certification in related health care fields (registered nurse, registered respiratory therapist, certified pulmonary function technician, etc.) are also desirable. A certified individual should be readily available to respond if needed.

4. Physicians are not required to be present during all tests. The physician ordering the test or a supervising laboratory physician may decide whether physician attendance at a specific test is required.

5. If a patient is on chronic oxygen therapy, oxygen should be given at their standard rate or as directed by a physician or a protocol.

Reasons for immediately stopping a 6MWT include the following: (1) chest pain, (2) intolerable dyspnea, (3) leg cramps, (4) staggering, (5) diaphoresis, and (6) pale or ashen appearance.

Technicians must be trained to recognize these problems and the appropriate responses. If a test is stopped for any of these reasons, the patient should sit or lie supine as appropriate depending on the severity of the event and the technician's assessment of the severity of the event and the risk of syncope. The following should be obtained based on the judgment of the technician: blood pressure, pulse rate, oxygen saturation, and a physician evaluation. Oxygen should be administered as appropriate.

Technical Aspects of the 6MWT

Location

The 6MWT should be performed indoors, along a long, flat, straight, enclosed corridor with a hard surface that is seldom traveled. If the weather is comfortable, the test may be performed outdoors. The walking course must be 30 m in length. A 100-ft hallway is, therefore, required. The length of the corridor should be marked every 3 m. The turnaround points should be marked with a cone (such as an orange traffic cone). A starting line, which marks the beginning and end of each 60-m lap, should be marked on the floor using brightly colored tape.

Rationale. A shorter corridor requires patients to take more time to reverse directions more often, reducing the 6MWD. Most studies have used a 30-m corridor, but some have used 20- or 50-m corridors.[52-55] A recent multicenter study found no significant effect of the length of straight courses ranging from 50 to 164 ft, but patients walked farther on continuous (oval) tracks (mean 92 ft farther).[54]

The use of a treadmill to determine the 6MWD might save space and allow constant monitoring during the exercise, but the use of a treadmill for 6-minute walk testing is not recommended. Patients are unable to pace themselves on a treadmill. In one study of patients with severe lung disease, the mean distance walked on the treadmill during 6 minutes (with the speed adjusted by the patients) was shorter by a mean of 14% when compared with the standard 6MWD using a 100-ft hallway.[57] The range of differences was wide, with patients walking between 400-1,300 ft on the treadmill who walked 1,200 ft in the hallway. Treadmill test results, therefore, are not interchangeable with corridor tests.

Required Equipment

1. Countdown timer (or stopwatch)
2. Mechanical lap counter
3. Two small cones to mark the turnaround points
4. A chair that can be easily moved along the walking course
5. Worksheets on a clipboard
6. A source of oxygen
7. Sphygmomanometer
8. Telephone
9. Automated electronic defibrillator

Patient Preparation

1. Comfortable clothing should be worn.
2. Appropriate shoes for walking should be worn.
3. Patients should use their usual walking aids during the test (cane, walker, etc.).
4. The patient's usual medical regimen should be continued.
5. A light meal is acceptable before early morning or early afternoon tests.

6. Patients should not have exercised vigorously within 2 hours of beginning the test.

Measurements

1. Repeat testing should be performed about the same time of day to minimize intraday variability.

2. A "warm-up" period before the test should not be performed.

3. The patient should sit at rest in a chair, located near the starting position, for at least 10 minutes before the test starts. During this time, check for contraindications, measure pulse and blood pressure, and make sure that clothing and shoes are appropriate. Complete the first portion of the worksheet (on page 135).

4. Pulse oximetry is optional. If it is performed, measure and record baseline heart rate and oxygen saturation (SpO_2) and follow manufacturer's instructions to maximize the signal and to minimize motion artifact.[56,57] Make sure the readings are stable before recording. Note pulse regularity and whether the oximeter signal quality is acceptable.

The rationale for measuring oxygen saturation is that although the distance is the primary outcome measure, improvement during serial evaluations may be manifest either by an increased distance or by reduced symptoms with the same distance walked.[39] The SpO_2 should not be used for constant monitoring during the exercise. The technician must not walk with the patient to observe the SpO_2. If worn during the walk, the pulse oximeter must be lightweight (less than 2 pounds), battery powered, and held in place (perhaps by a "fanny pack") so that the patient does not have to hold or stabilize it and so that stride is not affected. Many pulse oximeters have considerable motion artifact that prevents accurate readings during the walk.[57]

5. Have the patient stand and rate their baseline dyspnea and overall fatigue using the Borg scale (see table 2 for the Borg scale and instructions).[58]

6. Set the lap counter to zero and the timer to 6 minutes. Assemble all necessary equipment (lap counter, timer, clipboard, Borg Scale, worksheet) and move to the starting point.

Table 2	The Borg Scale
0	Nothing at all
0.5	Very, very slight (just noticeable)
1	Very slight
2	Slight (light)
3	Moderate
4	Somewhat severe
5	Severe (heavy)
6	
7	Very severe
8	
9	
10	Very, very severe (maximal)

This Borg scale should be printed on heavy paper (11 inches high and perhaps laminated) in 20-point type size. At the beginning of the 6-minute exercise, show the scale to the patient and ask the patient this: "Please grade your level of shortness of breath using this scale." Then ask this: "Please grade your level of fatigue using this scale."

At the end of the exercise, remind the patient of the breathing number that they chose before the exercise and ask the patient to grade their breathing level again. Then ask the patient to grade their level of fatigue, after reminding them of their grade before the exercise.

Please refer to the updated Borg Scale, which appears on page 136.

7. Instruct the patient as follows:

"The object of this test is to walk as far as possible for 6 minutes. You will walk back and forth in this hallway. Six minutes is a long time to walk, so you will be exerting yourself. You will probably get out of breath or become exhausted. You are permitted to slow down, to stop, and to rest as necessary. You may lean against the wall while resting, but resume walking as soon as you are able.

You will be walking back and forth around the cones. You should pivot briskly around the cones and continue back the other way without hesitation. Now I'm going to show you. Please watch the way I turn without hesitation."

Demonstrate by walking one lap yourself. Walk and pivot around a cone briskly.

"Are you ready to do that? I am going to use this counter to keep track of the number of laps you complete. I will click it each time you turn around at this starting line. Remember that the object is to walk AS FAR AS POSSIBLE for 6 minutes, but don't run or jog.

Start now, or whenever you are ready."

8. Position the patient at the starting line. You should also stand near the starting line during the test. Do not walk with the patient. As soon as the patient starts to walk, start the timer.

9. Do not talk to anyone during the walk. Use an even tone of voice when using the standard phrases of encouragement. Watch the patient. Do not get distracted and lose count of the laps. Each time the participant returns to the starting line, click the lap counter once (or mark the lap on the worksheet). Let the participant see you do it. Exaggerate the click using body language, like using a stopwatch at a race.

After the first minute, tell the patient the following (in even tones): "You are doing well. You have 5 minutes to go."

When the timer shows 4 minutes remaining, tell the patient the following: "Keep up the good work. You have 4 minutes to go."

When the timer shows 3 minutes remaining, tell the patient the following: "You are doing well. You are halfway done."

When the timer shows 2 minutes remaining, tell the patient the following: "Keep up the good work. You have only 2 minutes left."

When the timer shows only 1 minute remaining, tell the patient: "You are doing well. You have only 1 minute to go."

Do not use other words of encouragement (or body language) to speed up.

If the patient stops walking during the test and needs a rest, say this: "You can lean against the wall if you would like; then continue walking whenever you feel able." Do not stop the timer. If the patient stops before the 6 minutes are up and refuses to continue (or you decide that they should not continue), wheel the chair over for the patient to sit on, discontinue the walk, and note on the worksheet the distance, the time stopped, and the reason for stopping prematurely.

When the timer is 15 seconds from completion, say this: "In a moment I'm going to tell you to stop. When I do, just stop right where you are and I will come to you."

When the timer rings (or buzzes), say this: "Stop!" Walk over to the patient. Consider taking the chair if they look exhausted. Mark the spot where they stopped by placing a bean bag or a piece of tape on the floor.

10. Post-test: Record the postwalk Borg dyspnea and fatigue levels and ask this: "What, if anything, kept you from walking farther?"

11. If using a pulse oximeter, measure SpO_2 and pulse rate from the oximeter and then remove the sensor.

12. Record the number of laps from the counter (or tick marks on the worksheet).

13. Record the additional distance covered (the number of meters in the final partial lap) using the markers on the wall as distance guides. Calculate the total distance walked, rounding to the nearest meter, and record it on the worksheet.

14. Congratulate the patient on good effort and offer a drink of water.

Quality Assurance

Sources of Variability

There are many sources of 6MWD variability (see table 3). The sources of variability caused by the test procedure itself should be controlled as much as possible. This is done by following the standards found in this document and by using a quality-assurance program.

Table 3   6MWD Sources of Variability
Factors Reducing the 6MWD
Shorter height
Older age
Higher body weight
Female sex
Impaired cognition
A shorter corridor (more turns)
Pulmonary disease (COPD, asthma, cystic fibrosis, interstitial lung disease)
Cardiovascular disease (angina, MI, CHF, stroke, TIA, PVD, AAI)
Musculoskeletal disorders (arthritis, ankle, knee, or hip injuries, muscle wasting, etc.)
Factors Increasing the 6MWD
Taller height (longer legs)
Male sex
High motivation
A patient who has previously performed the test
Medication for a disabling disease taken just before the test
Oxygen supplementation in patients with exercise-induced hypoxemia

Definition of abbreviations: COPD = chronic obstructive pulmonary disease; 6MWD = 6-minute walking distance.

Practice Tests

A practice test is not needed in most clinical settings but should be considered. If a practice test is done, wait for at least one hour before the second test and report the highest 6MWD as the patient's 6MWD baseline.

Rationale. The 6MWD is only slightly higher for a second 6MWT performed a day later. The mean reported increase ranges from 0 to 17%.[23,27,40,41,54-59] A multicenter study of 470 highly motivated patients with severe COPD performed two 6MWTs one day apart, and on average, the 6MWD was only 66 ft (5.8%) higher on the second day.[54]

Performance (without an intervention) usually reaches a plateau after two tests done within a week.[8,60] The training effect may be due to improved coordination, finding optimal stride length, and overcoming anxiety. The possibility of a practice or training effect from tests repeated after more than a month has not been studied or reported; however, it is likely that the effect of training wears off (does not persist) after a few weeks.

Technician Training and Experience

Technicians who perform 6MWTs should be trained using the standard protocol and then supervised for several tests before performing them alone. They should also have completed cardiopulmonary resuscitation training.

Rationale. One multicenter study of older people found that after correction for many other factors, two of the technicians had mean 6MWDs that were approximately 7% lower than the other two sites.[31]

Encouragement

Only the standardized phrases for encouragement (as specified previously here) must be used during the test.

Rationale. Encouragement significantly increases the distance walked.[42] Reproducibility for tests with and without encouragement is similar. Some studies have used encouragement every 30 seconds, every minute, or every 2 minutes. We have chosen every minute and standard phrases. Some studies[53] have instructed patients to walk as fast as possible. Although larger mean 6MWDs may be obtained thereby, we recommend that such phrases not be used, as they emphasize initial speed at the expense of earlier fatigue and possible excessive cardiac stress in some patients with heart disease.

Supplemental Oxygen

If oxygen supplementation is needed during the walks and serial tests are planned (after an intervention other than oxygen therapy), then during all walks by that patient oxygen should be delivered in the same way with the same flow. If the flow must be increased during subsequent visits due to worsening gas exchange, this should be noted on the worksheet and considered during interpretation of the change noted in 6MWD. The type of oxygen delivery device should also be noted on the report: for instance, the patient carried liquid oxygen or pushed or pulled an oxygen tank, the delivery was pulsed or continuous, or a technician walked behind the patient with the oxygen source (not recommended). Measurements of pulse and SpO_2 should be made after waiting at least 10 minutes after any change in oxygen delivery.

Rationale. For patients with COPD or interstitial lung disease, oxygen supplementation increases the 6MWD.[17,59,61,63] Carrying a portable gas container (but not using it for supplemental oxygen) reduced the mean 6MWD by 14% in one study of patients with severe respiratory disability, but using the container to deliver supplemental oxygen during the exercise increased the mean 6MWD by 20-35%.[59]

Medications

The type of medication, dose, and number of hours taken before the test should be noted.

Rationale. Significant improvement in the distance walked, or the dyspnea scale, after administration of bronchodilators has been demonstrated in patients with COPD,[62,63] as well as cardiovascular medications in patients with heart failure.[19]

Interpretation

Most 6MWTs will be done before and after intervention, and the primary question to be answered after both tests have been completed is whether the patient has experienced a clinically significant improvement. With a good quality-assurance program, with patients tested by the same technician, and after one or two practice tests, short-term reproducibility of the 6MWD is excellent.[37] It is not known whether it is best for clinical purposes to express change in 6MWD as (1) an absolute value, (2) a percentage change, or (3) a change in the percentage of predicted value. Until further research is available, we recommend that change in 6MWD be expressed as an absolute value (e.g., the patient walked 50 m farther).

A statistically significant mean increase in 6MWD in a group of study participants is often much less than a clinically significant increase in an individual patient. In one study of 112 patients (half of them women) with stable, severe COPD, the smallest difference in 6MWD that was associated with a noticeable clinical difference in the patients' perception of exercise performance was a mean of 54 m (95% confidence interval, 37-71 m).[64] This study suggests that for individual patients with COPD, an improvement of more than 70 m in the 6MWD after an intervention is necessary to be 95% confident that the improvement was significant. In an observational study of 45 older patients with heart failure, the smallest difference in 6MWD that was associated with a noticeable difference in their global rating of worsening was a mean of 43 m.[20] The 6MWD was more responsive to deterioration than to improvement in heart failure symptoms.

Reported Mean Changes in 6MWD After Interventions

Supplemental oxygen (4 L/min) during exercise in patients with COPD or interstitial lung disease increased mean 6MWD by approximately 95 m (36%) in one study.[59] Patients taking an inhaled corticosteroid experienced a mean 33 m (8%) increase in 6MWD in an international COPD study.[16] Patients with COPD in a study of the effects of exercise and diaphragmatic strength training experienced a mean increase in 6MWD of 50 m (20%).[65] Lung volume reduction surgery in patients with very severe COPD has been reported to increase 6MWD by a mean of 55 m (20%).[13]

Cardiac rehabilitation in patients referred with various heart diseases increased 6MWD by a mean of 170 m (15%) in a recent study.[66] In 25 older patients with heart failure, an angiotensin-converting enzyme inhibitor medication (50 mg captopril per day) improved 6MWD a mean of 64 m (39%) compared with a mean increase of only 8% in those receiving a placebo.[19]

Interpreting Single Measurements of Functional Status

Optimal reference equations from healthy population-based samples using standardized 6MWT methods are not yet available. In one study, the median 6MWD was approximately 580 m for 117 healthy men and 500 m for 173 healthy women.[50] A mean 6MWD of 630 m was reported by another study of 51 healthy older adults.[55] Differences in the population sampled, type and frequency of encouragement, corridor length, and number of practice tests may account for reported differences in mean 6MWD in healthy persons. Age, height, weight, and sex independently affect the 6MWD in healthy adults; therefore, these factors should be taken into consideration when interpreting the results of single measurements made to determine functional status. We encourage investigators to publish reference equations for healthy persons using the previously mentioned standardized procedures.

A low 6MWD is nonspecific and nondiagnostic. When the 6MWD is reduced, a thorough search for the cause of the impairment is warranted. The following tests may then be helpful: pulmonary function, cardiac function, ankle-arm index, muscle strength, nutritional status, orthopedic function, and cognitive function.

Conclusions

The 6MWT is a useful measure of functional capacity targeted at people with at least moderately severe impairment. The test has been widely used for preoperative and postoperative evaluation and for measuring the response to therapeutic interventions for pulmonary and cardiac disease. These guidelines provide a standardized approach to performing the 6MWT. The committee hopes that these guidelines will encourage further research into the 6MWT and allow direct comparisons among different studies.

This statement was developed by the ATS Committee on Proficiency Standards for Clinical Pulmonary Function Laboratories.

Members of the committee are
Robert O. Crapo, MD, Chair*
Richard Casaburi, PhD, MD
Allan L. Coates, MD
Paul L. Enright, MD
Neil R. MacIntyre, MD
Roy T. McKay, PhD
Douglas Johnson, MD
Jack S. Wanger, MS
R. Jorge Zeballos, MD*

Ad Hoc Committee members are
Vera Bittner, MD
Carl Mottram, RRT
*Writing Committee members

Appendix Form

The following elements should be present on the 6MWT worksheet and report:

Lap counter: _____

Patient name: _____ Patient ID #: _____

Walk #: _____ Tech ID: _____ Date: _____

Gender: M F   Age: _____ Race: _____ Height: _____ ft _____ in. _____ meters

Weight: _____ lbs _____ kg   Blood pressure: _____/_____

Medications taken before the test (dose and time): _____

Supplemental oxygen during the test: No   Yes, flow _____ L/min, type _____

	Baseline	End of test
Time	_____:_____	_____:_____
Heart rate	_____	_____
Dyspnea	_____	_____ (Borg scale)
Fatigue	_____	_____ (Borg scale)
SpO$_2$	_____%	_____%

Stopped or paused before 6 minutes? No Yes reason: _____

Other symptoms at end of exercise: angina dizziness hip, leg, or calf pain

Number of laps: _____ (x 60 meters) + final partial lap: _____ meters = _____

Total distance walked in 6 minutes: _____ meters

Predicted distance: _____ meters   Percent predicted: _____%

Tech comments: _____

_____

Interpretation (including comparison with a preintervention 6MWD): _____

_____

Reprinted, by permission, from American Thoracic Society, 2002, "ATS Statement: Guidelines for the six-minute walk test," *American Journal of Respiratory and Critical Care Medicine* 166: 111-117.

The Borg RPE Scale

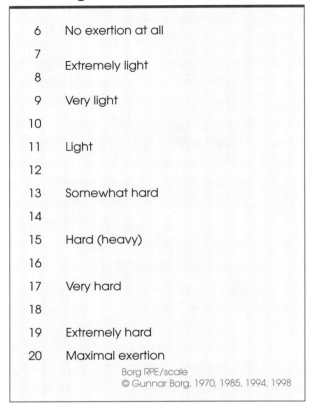

6	No exertion at all
7	
	Extremely light
8	
9	Very light
10	
11	Light
12	
13	Somewhat hard
14	
15	Hard (heavy)
16	
17	Very hard
18	
19	Extremely hard
20	Maximal exertion

Borg RPE/scale
© Gunnar Borg, 1970, 1985, 1994, 1998

Reprinted, by permission, from G. Borg, 1998, *Borg's perceived exertion pain scale* (Champaign, IL: Human Kinetics), 47.

appendix d

Clinical Competency Guidelines for Pulmonary Rehabilitation Professionals

American Association of Cardiovascular and Pulmonary Rehabilitation Position Statement

Pulmonary Clinical Competencies Working Group:

Douglas R. Southard, PhD, MPH, Chair*
Lawrence P. Cahalin, MA, PT†
Brian W. Carlin, MD‡
Mollyn Cales, RN§
Valerie K. McLeod, RRT //
Kathleen Morris, RN, MS, RRT¶
Edgar A. Normandin, PhD, PT#
Jane Reardon, RN**
Andrew L. Ries, MD, MPH††
Alexandra J. Sciaky, PT, CCS‡‡

From the *Virginia Polytechnic Institute and State University, Blacksburg, Virginia; †Massachusetts General Hospital, Boston, Massachusetts; ‡Alle-gheny General Hospital, Pittsburgh, Pennsylvania; §Southern West Virginia Clinic, Beckley, West Virginia; //McLaren Regional Medical Center, Flint, Michigan; ¶St. Helena Hospital, Deer Park, California; #St. Francis Hospital and Medical Center, Hartford, Connecticut; **Hartford Hospital, Hartford, Connecticut; ††University of California, San Diego Medical Center, San Diego, California; and ‡‡University of Michigan Medical Center, Ann Arbor, Michigan.

Address for correspondence: Douglas R. Southard, PhD, MPH, Virginia Tech, 103 War Memorial Hall, Blacksburg, VA 24061-0351.

Reprinted, by permission, from D.R. Southard, et al. 1995, "Clinical competency guidelines for pulmonary rehabilitation professionals: American Association of Cardiovascular and Pulmonary Rehabilitation position statement," *J Cardiopulm Rehabil* 15: 173-178.

Definition and Purpose

This document presents an outline of the clinical competencies recommended for those providing comprehensive services in pulmonary rehabilitation. It is assumed that individuals wishing to provide such services should possess a common core of professional and clinical competencies regardless of their academic discipline. Services characteristic of a comprehensive pulmonary rehabilitation program include a multidisciplinary assessment leading to the development of an integrated treatment plan, including patient education, exercise training, psychosocial support, and follow-up. Practitioners may also serve as case managers to provide coordination of services. Individuals who commonly provide such comprehensive services include respiratory care practitioners, nurses, physical therapists, occupational therapists, exercise physiologists, and others.

In addition to the general guidelines outlined in this paper, pulmonary rehabilitation professionals should be aware of state limitations of practice acts and techniques of legal risk management as they apply to assessment, intervention, and follow-up. They should also demonstrate understanding of infection control procedures, including implications of Occupational Safety and Health Administration (OSHA) bloodborne pathogen standards and the application of universal precautions to clinical procedures.

Because of the growing recognition of the benefits of pulmonary rehabilitation for patients with chronic obstructive pulmonary disease, the applications of rehabilitation principles to patients with other lung diseases are increasingly being developed and refined. These include but are not limited to individuals with asthma, cystic fibrosis, lung transplantation, interstitial/restrictive lung diseases, and ventilator dependency. This document does not specifically address these other patient populations, but does recognize the potential value of rehabilitation for all patients with chronic lung diseases and the need for further research and development.

By itself, this document conveys no approval, endorsements, or certification of either pulmonary rehabilitation professionals or their programs. Rather, it identifies and promotes common practice expectations. In doing so, the document may also serve as a self-evaluation tool for practitioners to identify continuing education needs.

During the course of its development, this manuscript underwent reviews by the American Association of Cardiovascular and Pulmonary Rehabilitation (AACVPR) Board of Directors and the Publications Committee. The document is organized into three major clinical process categories (Assessment, Intervention, and Outcome Evaluation/Follow-up) and six content categories.

Competency Guidelines

I. Assessment

A. Pathophysiology and Comorbidity

1. Demonstrates a thorough knowledge of pulmonary and cardiovascular anatomy, physiology, and pathophysiology including common pulmonary and cardiovascular conditions limiting or otherwise influencing physical activity, symptom management, respiratory and chest physical therapy, dietary modification, smoking cessation, and stress management.

2. Demonstrates an understanding of pulmonary and cardiovascular diagnostic techniques, medical and pharmacologic management, and the normal/abnormal pulmonary and cardiovascular responses to exercise.

3. Recognizes comorbid conditions including metabolic (e.g., diabetes, obesity), musculoskeletal (e.g., hip or knee dysfunction, osteoporosis, arthritis), and other conditions (e.g., gastroesophageal reflux with chronic aspiration, hiatal hernia, sinusitis/rhinitis, alcoholism, sleep disturbances, etc.) that may influence the prescription of physical activity, dietary intake, ventilatory muscle training, breathing retraining, smoking cessation, or stress management.

4. Recognizes the effects of environmental factors, medication usage, and supplemental oxygen usage on the pathophysiology, treatment, and natural history of the disease process.

5. Demonstrates a level of understanding of general anatomy, physiology, and pathophysiology equivalent to a semester length course each in anatomy/physiology and pathophysiology.

6. Recognizes the appropriate time frame for physiologic changes to occur as well as how physiologic responses to one rehabilitation modality (i.e., breathing retraining) may influence the individual's response to other interventions (i.e., stair climbing, etc.).

B. Professional Communication

1. Obtains records regarding medical/health history to include diagnoses and therapeutic course.

2. Informs patient̶
   responsibilities w
   professional eth
   including a leg̶
   sent process, ̶
   tiality, appro̶
   patient info
   patients of t̶
   the extent provideu ̶
   sions regarding acceptance ̶
   medical treatment.

3. Consults with referring physician and other health care team members to determine the need for additional assessments.

4. Prepares a summary of patient evaluation using multidisciplinary assessment data.

5. Develops, with active patient participation, a comprehensive plan of rehabilitation, including the establishment of reasonable and measurable goals.

6. Documents assessment and treatment plans in appropriate clinical formats.

7. Develops a system of communicating the results of the comprehensive patient evaluation to the patient and primary care and/or referring physician.

C. Patient Education and Training

1. Gathers historical and physical evidence relevant to determining both non-modifiable (age and sex) and modifiable/treatable factors (e.g., smoking, occupational and other environmental irritant exposure, excess alcohol intake, altitude at which patient resides, respiratory rate and depth, infections, physical and emotional stressors, underlying connective tissue disorder, alpha-1 antitrypsin deficiency, responses to bronchodilator therapy, etc.).

2. Screens for appropriate nutritional intake and eating habits.

3. Assesses need for immunizations (i.e., Pneumovax influenza vaccine).

4. Explains the interaction of pulmonary risk factors with each other (smoking, obesity, environmental irritants, occupational exposures, allergies, etc.) and their possible impact on disease progression.

̶ appropriate goals for
̶s needing behavior modifi-
for improving coping skills.

̶rinciples of adult learning
̶essing client's learning needs.

̶ information regarding edu-
̶ and literacy level, the presence
̶al or hearing impairments, and
age or cultural barriers.

̶sses the patient's and family's
̶wledge of pulmonary anatomy,
̶ysiology, and pathophysiology.

9. Assesses for the use of prescription and nonprescription medications that might have an adverse effect on airway function, physical activity, or cardiovascular and pulmonary symptoms.

10. Assesses for current and previous use of tobacco products, attempts to quit, and current level of psychological and chemical (nicotine) dependency.

11. Assesses patient's ability to effectively administer metered dose inhalers, nebulizers, oxygen, and other prescribed medications and treatments as well as for the presence of medication abuse.

12. Assesses patient's frequency of air or other high altitude travel, and level of understanding regarding its effects on pulmonary function.

13. Assesses patient's need for bronchial hygiene techniques including percussion, vibration, postural drainage, and controlled coughing, and identifies resources for providing such care.

14. Assesses patient's breathing pattern and need for breathing retraining and other respiratory muscle exercises.

D. Exercise

1. Assesses physical activity patterns as well as vocational and avocational preferences (past and present).

2. Interprets the information obtained from the invasive or noninvasive assessment of pulmonary and cardiovascular capacity that may include appropriate modes (tests of pulmonary function and gas exchange, blood gases, treadmill, bicycle ergometer, walk test, etc.), protocols (incremental, steady state exercise, etc.), and monitoring (heart rate, blood pressure, oximetry, electrocardiography,

ratings of perceived exertion and breathlessness, respiratory rate, ventilatory muscle strength and endurance, arterial blood gases, etc.) to accommodate patients with specific needs, disabilities, or disorders as well as to assess patient needs and ensure patient safety.

3. Demonstrates an understanding of pulmonary and cardiovascular findings (ventilatory muscle strength and endurance, pulmonary function, bronchial hygiene, and supplementary oxygen needs, etc.), as well as body composition, strength, endurance, and flexibility in the assessment of the functional capacity necessary to meet the demands of vocational, avocational, and activities of daily living (ADLs).

4. Demonstrates an understanding of the physiologic response to physical activity as well as the various tests/measurements used to develop the exercise prescription (i.e., ventilatory performance, dyspnea indexes, gas exchange abnormalities, respiratory rate, heart rate, pulmonary reserve, metabolic equivalents (METS), ratings of perceived exertion (RPE), blood gases, lactate levels, and anaerobic threshold, etc.).

5. Demonstrates an understanding of the effects of environmental factors (i.e., elevated pollen count, altitude, humidity and temperature), medication usage (i.e., nebulizer), or supplemental oxygen that limit or otherwise influence exercise performance.

E. Psychosocial

1. Utilizes active listening and behavioral observation skills in health counseling.

2. Assesses for impairments in interpersonal functioning and level of family and social support (quality and quantity).

3. Evaluates stress level in terms of life events, level of self-reported emotional distress, level of stress-related psychophysiologic responses (i.e., excessive muscle tension) to chronic illness, and physiologic responses (dyspnea, elevations in heart rate, blood pressure, and respiration) to daily stressors.

4. Identifies appropriate psychosocial adaptation to illness and screens for the presence of maladaptive behaviors and psychopathology (i.e., depression, anger, anxiety/panic, excessive grief reaction to losses, decreased symptom management skills, over-dependence on others, etc.).

5. Assesses for impairments in sexual activity in relation to the disease state.

6. Demonstrates an understanding of the psychosocial issues affecting adherence to various intervention strategies and the development of an integrated treatment plan.

7. Assesses adequacy of patient and family resources (i.e., financial status, insurance coverage, etc.) to complete rehabilitation plan.

8. Assesses need for referral to appropriate community services, support groups, and follow-up care.

F. Emergency Procedures

1. Demonstrates knowledge and skills appropriate for managing pulmonary, cardiovascular, and other types of emergencies that may be encountered with patients undergoing assessment procedures. The minimum requirements are current certification in cardiopulmonary resuscitation, (i.e., Health Care Provider Basic Cardiac Life Support, [BCLS]; American Heart Association or equivalent).

2. Assesses patient's and family's level of knowledge and skills in emergency procedures.

II. Intervention

A. Pathophysiology and Comorbidity

1. Demonstrates an understanding of pulmonary, cardiovascular, and common metabolic and musculoskeletal conditions in terms of their influence on the implementation, monitoring, and adjustment of interventions.

B. Professional Communication

1. Communicates and documents the delivery of care to patients. This includes recording the patient's responses to treatment, as well as the patient's adherence/nonadherence to prescribed protocols and lifestyle recommendations.

2. Documents in a timely and accurate manner any clinical findings that require medical follow-up for reasons of patient safety and success of treatment.

3. Demonstrates effective interpersonal skills with patients, the patients' significant others, and other health care providers who are involved in the patient's health care.

4. Maintains confidentiality and observes patient's personal and cultural value system within the context of clinical responsibilities and medicolegal norms.

5. Develops a timely and consistent system for status reports to the primary care and/or referring physician.

6. Refers to other health care professionals as appropriate.

C. Patient Education and Training

1. Uses basic educational principles, theories of learning, and methods of counseling, as well as knowledge of specific behavioral modification techniques used for breathing retraining, smoking cessation, and dietary modification.

2. Monitors clinical symptoms and laboratory data during the course of treatment that may indicate important changes relating to disease progression or lifestyle management. This would include an understanding of realistic expectations for improvement as well as circumstances during treatment that should prompt referral of the patient for consultation by specialized health professionals. Clinical domains to be monitored include: heart rate, respiratory rate, oxygen saturation, medication usage, weight loss/gain, presence of reflux, breath sounds (i.e., for secretions, etc.), dyspnea/exertion level, blood pressure, smoking status, diabetic control, and electrocardiography as indicated.

3. Develops an integrated education/ training program, using a multidisciplinary approach, consisting of exercise, dyspnea management, activities of daily living training, panic control, smoking cessation, and stress management.

4. Provides patient training regarding appropriate use of medications and potential for side effects.

5. Instructs and counsels patients using a variety of methods, strategies, materials, and technologies helpful in promoting behavior change.

6. Adjusts teaching to accommodate individual patient needs and limitations.

7. Enables patients to acquire the perspective, knowledge, and skills necessary to independently maintain optimal health after discharge from pulmonary rehabilitation care.

8. Teaches and counsels patients regarding travel and altitude (including air travel), particularly for patients requiring supplemental oxygen therapy.

9. Provides and teaches individualized respiratory care exercises to patients. These programs may include: percussion, postural drainage, vibration, controlled coughing and breathing exercises, and use of oxygen (i.e., hours of usage, liter flow at rest and with exercise).

10. Demonstrates ability to counsel regarding durable power of attorney for health care services and advanced directives.

D. Exercise

1. Develops an exercise prescription, in collaboration with the physician who will safely and effectively guide the patient toward optimal restoration and maintenance of functional capacity both on site and at home.

2. Leads, monitors, and supervises individual and group therapeutic exercise sessions appropriate to patients with varying degrees of pulmonary and cardiovascular disease.

3. Demonstrates competence to determine when ECG telemetry is indicated during exercise sessions.

4. Explains hazards of high-risk patient behaviors during exercise training (i.e., exceeding targets for dyspnea or exertional hypoxemia, exercising in excessively hot or cold weather, etc.), and how these may be reduced through patient training, supervision, and appropriate monitoring techniques.

5. Demonstrates proper techniques for performing patient's preferred avocational physical activities (i.e., golf,

shopping, etc.) and for correcting faults in patient's technique.

E. Psychosocial

1. Suggests self-help techniques, materials, and resources, and/or refers the patient to mental health professionals, support groups, community, and home care services as appropriate.

2. Provides supportive counsel to individuals experiencing mild-moderate psychological distress (i.e., depression, anxiety/panic, anger, etc.).

3. Explains and promotes appropriate relaxation skills and other stress management techniques.

4. Involves family members or significant others as appropriate in counseling to enhance social support.

5. Provides information, if needed, about techniques that can minimize disease-related limitations on sexual activity.

F. Emergency Procedures

1. Maintains an emergency response capability for pulmonary rehabilitation exercise programs. This should include appropriate equipment in the exercise area along with an understanding of staff roles and the specific steps needed for various pulmonary, cardiovascular, and other emergency situations.

2. Demonstrates knowledge of medicolegal and licensing authority issues that mandate specific roles for different professionals in the making of medical decisions and in the delivery of emergency care (i.e., licensed authority to perform advanced cardiac life support [ACLS]).

3. Encourages family members to enroll in a basic cardiopulmonary resuscitation (CPR) course and identify community emergency services.

III. Outcome Evaluation and Follow-Up

A. Pathophysiology and Comorbidity

1. Evaluates whether the patient's rehabilitation program was adjusted appropriately and medical therapy provided to address any pulmonary, cardiovascular, or other medical conditions (e.g., diabetes, obesity, arthritis, etc.) that

may have adversely affected the desired rehabilitation outcomes.

B. Professional Communication

1. Completes discharge summary describing client's progression in rehabilitation program in terms of: symptom changes, commitment to lifestyle changes, exercise responses, identified barriers and possible solutions to noncompliant behaviors, and achievement of personal goals (return of lost abilities such as shopping, golf, bowling, etc.) leading to an enhanced quality of life. Summary to be sent to referring physician and team members as needed.

2. Communicates to patient the degree of success in completing goals and steps that must be taken to maintain/improve gains.

3. Facilitates ongoing self-care, home-care, follow-up, and support services after discharge from pulmonary rehabilitation care.

C. Patient Education and Training

1. Reassesses patient prognosis as it relates to the risk factor profile (occupational exposure, smoking, etc.).

2. Develops long-term plan to improve risk factor profile, involving both patient and family.

3. Evaluates follow-through in medication and oxygen usage and self-administration techniques.

4. Determines if client was successful in returning to desired vocational, avocational, and/or recreational activities.

5. Evaluates if interventions undertaken to accommodate the patient's verbal or written impairments, educational limitations, and visual or hearing defects have been successful.

6. Reassesses patient's self-care regimen to include activities of daily living, pulmonary hygiene skills, medication management, social/community support, and appropriate ongoing medical care, and adjusts accordingly.

D. Exercise

1. Assists client to reevaluate physical activity patterns and preferences regard-

ing specific exercise modalities (bicycle vs. treadmill, etc.).

2. Reevaluates cardiopulmonary capacity for exercise, determines compliance with initial home exercise program, and updates exercise prescription and treatment regimen.

3. Reevaluates pulmonary function, cardiovascular status, body composition, strength, endurance, and flexibility in terms of ability to meet the demands of vocational, avocational, and activities of daily living (ADLs).

E. Psychosocial

1. Reassesses stress levels and modifies treatment plan accordingly.

2. Evaluates if mental health consultation and/or referrals to support groups, community, and home care services were performed based on needs determined at the initial assessment and progress through rehabilitation program.

3. Evaluates client's progress in achieving desired goals related to sexual activity.

4. Reassesses effectiveness of social support and enhances support network as needed.

F. Emergency Procedures

1. Demonstrates capability to evaluate the patient's and family's ability to monitor for signs and symptoms of respiratory infection and impending respiratory failure.

2. Modifies interventions when potential safety hazards are discovered or specific problems identified to increase margins of safety.

3. Reassesses the client's and family's knowledge of emergency procedures (i.e., CPR).

Acknowledgments

The Writing Group thanks John Hodgkin, MD, Kevin Ryan, RRT, the AACVPR Board of Directors and Publications Committee, and other rehabilitation professionals for their guidance and feedback regarding earlier drafts of this document.

appendix e

Examples of Pulmonary Rehabilitation Programs That Meet 2, 3, and 5 Days a Week

Typical Twice-Weekly, Eight-Week Program Outpatient Pulmonary Rehabilitation Schedule*

Week 1: Nutritional and Respiratory Assessments	
Appointment date: _____	Appointment time: _____

Week 2: Tuesday 01/21/04 1:30 P.M.	Thursday 01/23/04 1:30 P.M.
1:30-2:30 Orientation to program; education session on lung disease 2:30-4:00 Supervised exercise	1:30-2:30 Breathing retraining and inhaler use 2:30-4:00 Supervised exercise

Week 3: Tuesday 01/28/04 1:30 P.M.	Thursday 01/30/04 1:30 P.M.
1:30-2:30 Lung medications 2:30-4:00 Supervised exercise	1:30-2:30 Medications part 2 or review 2:30-4:00 Supervised exercise

Week 4: Tuesday 02/04/04 1:30 P.M.	Thursday 02/06/04 1:30 P.M.
1:30-2:30 Food, lungs, and their relationship 2:30-4:00 Supervised exercise	1:30-2:30 What are these tests for? 2:30-4:00 Supervised exercise

Week 5: Tuesday 02/11/04 1:30 P.M.	Thursday 02/13/04 1:30 P.M.
1:30-2:30 Energy conservation 2:30-4:00 Supervised exercise and stairs	1:30-2:30 Preventing infection 2:30-4:00 Supervised exercise and stairs

Week 6: Tuesday 02/18/04 1:30 P.M.	Thursday 02/20/04 1:30 P.M.
1:30-2:30 Improving the immune system and relaxation techniques 2:30-4:00 Supervised exercise and stairs	1:30-2:00 Relaxation and panic control 2:00-2:45 Living with lung disease 2:45-4:00 Supervised exercise

Week 7: Tuesday 02/25/04 1:30 P.M.	Thursday 02/27/04 1:30 P.M.
1:30-2:30 Community resources 2:30-4:00 Supervised exercise	Individually scheduled 6-minute walk tests* 1:30-2:30 Benefits of exercise 2:30-4:00 Supervised exercise

Week 8: Tuesday 03/04/04 1:30 P.M.	Thursday 03/06/04 1:30 P.M.
1:30-2:00 Taking pulmonary rehabilitation home 2:00-3:30 Supervised exercise	1:30-2:00 Program evaluation and graduation 2:00-3:30 Supervised exercise

Three-Day Pulmonary Rehabilitation Program*

Monday, Wednesday, Friday; 2-hour format

Check-in: 10 minutes

Warm-up and breathing retraining: 10 minutes

Weight training and stretching: 20 minutes

Aerobic training (ambulation on treadmill or level surface): 20 minutes

Biking aerobic training (bike ergometer with arms and legs, legs only, or arm ergometry—patient may do one of the bike choices or a combination that would total 20 minutes): 20 minutes

Cool-down: 10 minutes

Education: 30 minutes

Five-Day Pulmonary Rehabilitation Program*

Monday through Friday, 4-hour format

Check-in: 10 minutes

Circuit weight training: 20 minutes

Pulmonary hygiene (may include chest physical therapy, nebulizer, instruction in inhaler use, or breathing retraining): 30 minutes

Floor exercise (breathing retraining, muscle toning, stretching): 60 minutes

Aerobic training (ambulation on treadmill or level surface): 30 minutes

Biking aerobic training (bike ergometer with arms and legs, legs only, or arm ergometry—patient may do one of the bike choices or a combination that would total 30 minutes): 30 minutes

Education: 60 minutes

* Make sure there is a 5-10 minute rest break between each activity.

Example of a Typical Pulmonary Rehabilitation Facility

Facility Areas

- Waiting or reception area
- Pulmonary rehabilitation administrative assistant's office
- Pulmonary rehabilitation program coordinator's office
- Storage room
- Classroom

Description of Areas

- Pulmonary rehabilitation waiting or reception area and office

  Equipment includes desks, computer, chairs for patients, staff equipment and supplies, and public telephone.

- Pulmonary rehabilitation classroom

  Equipment includes patient notebooks and supplies appropriate for pulmonary rehabilitation training, tables, chairs, whiteboard, and VCR.

- Gymnasium

  Equipment includes exercise equipment appropriate for pulmonary rehabilitation exercise sessions (e.g., indoor level-surface track, treadmills, stationary bikes, rowing machines, stair stepper, treadmills, floor exercise space, and weights) as well as blood pressure cuffs, stethoscopes, supplemental oxygen sources, pulse oximeters, and emergency equipment.

appendix g

Pulmonary Rehabilitation Skills and Competency Assessment

Employee Name: _____

Pulmonary Rehabilitation Skills and Competency Assessment Exercise Component: Demonstrates under-standing and use of exercise principles and modalities, the ability to instruct patients with chronic lung disease.

Self-Evaluation Key:
2 = feels competent
1 = needs review
0 = not applicable

Plan If Needed Key:
L = learn skill or info
P = practice skill or technique
V = validate knowledge

Evaluator Assessment Key:
2 = verbally explains or demonstrates
1 = needs review
0 = not applicable

	Self-Evaluation	Comments/Plan	Evaluator Assessment
1. Able to assess and instruct patients according to their age-specific needs and cultural beliefs			
2. Identifies patient's learning style and barriers to learning and incorporates them when working with the patient			
3. Complies with HIPPA and respects the patient's rights, confidentiality, and individual needs			
4. Knows the emergency protocol, how to use the emergency equipment and supplies, how to complete a clinical event form, and when to notify the patient's physician(s) and the PR medical director			
5. Performs 6-minute timed distance walk test, completes the calculations for the exercise prescription, and documents correctly			
6. Able to develop an individualized exercise prescription based on 6-minute walk test, orthopedic and other comorbid conditions, pain, etc.			
7. Able to describe common exercise limitations that will require modifications for the exercise modalities			
8. Able to provide verbal and manual cueing for breathing techniques and pursed-lip breathing/diaphragmatic breathing, and incorporated them into the exercise regime			
9. Monitors patient's oxygen saturation and titrates supplemental oxygen, as needed			

	Self-Evaluation	Comments/Plan	Evaluator Assessment
10. Able to identify the proper use of appropriate oxygen device to maintain an oxygen saturation >90-92% (oxymizer, nonrebreather mask, etc.)			
11. Correctly uses equipment and instructs patient appropriately, monitoring for patient safety			
12. Instructs and progresses exercises in a safe manner and monitors patient's tolerance			
13. Demonstrates use of graded exercise techniques and interval training			
14. Able to use and instruct patient in the correct exercises and techniques for universal weight equipment			
15. Instructs patient and family in the home exercise program (HEP) and has them keep an exercise log			
16. Maintains and cleans equipment according to policies and procedures and checks inventory weekly			

Section II: Pulmonary Rehabilitation Competency Assessment

Self-Evaluation Key:
2 = feels competent
1 = needs review
0 = not applicable

Evaluator Assessment Key:
2 = verbally explains or demonstrates
1 = needs review
0 = not applicable

	Self-Evaluation	Comments/Plan	Evaluator Assessment

(continued)

Competency adheres to hospital policy, community standards, and professional requirements as delineated by but not limited to:

a. Laws and Regulations relating to the Standards of Practice of Physical Therapy, State of California, Department of Consumer Affairs, PT Examining Committee
b. General Guidelines for Professional Conduct and Code of Ethics, American Physical Therapy Association

Overall Summary

_____

_____

_____

Employee signature: _____

Date: _____

Evaluator signature: _____

Date: _____

references

Chapter 1

1. American College of Chest Physicians and American Association of Cardiovascular and Pulmonary Rehabilitation Guidelines Panel. 1997. Pulmonary rehabilitation: Joint ACCP/AACVPR evidence-based guidelines. *Chest* 112: 1363-1396.

2. Fabbri, L.M., and Hurd, S.S. 2003. Global strategy for the diagnosis, management, and prevention of COPD: 2003 update. *Eur Respir J* 22: 1-2.

3. National Emphysema Treatment Trial Research Group. 2003. A randomized trial comparing lung-volume-reduction surgery with medical therapy for severe emphysema. *N Engl J Med* 348 (21): 2059-2073.

4. American College of Chest Physicians and American Association of Cardiovascular and Pulmonary Rehabilitation Guidelines Panel. 1997. Pulmonary rehabilitation: Joint ACCP/AACVPR evidence-based guidelines. *J Cardiopulmon Rehabil* 17: 371-405.

5. American Association of Cardiovascular and Pulmonary Rehabilitation. 1998. *Guidelines for pulmonary rehabilitation programs,* 2nd ed. Champaign, IL: Human Kinetics.

6. Ries, A.L. 1990. Position paper of the American Association of Cardiovascular and Pulmonary Rehabilitation: Scientific basis of pulmonary rehabilitation. *J Cardiopulm Rehabil* 10: 418-441.

7. Hodgkin, J.E. 2000. Benefits and the future of pulmonary rehabilitation. In *Pulmonary rehabilitation: Guidelines to success,* 3rd ed. Edited by J.E. Hodgkin, B.R. Celli, and G.L. Connors, 693. Philadelphia: Lippincott Williams & Wilkins.

8. Hodgkin, J.E. 1996. Benefits of pulmonary rehabilitation. In *Pulmonary rehabilitation: Lung biology in health and disease,* vol. 91. Edited by A.P. Fishman, 33-46. New York: Marcel Dekker.

9. American Thoracic Society. 1981. Position statement on pulmonary rehabilitation. *Am Rev Respir Dis* 1136: 663.

10. Fishman, A.P. 1994. Pulmonary rehabilitation research: NIH workshop summary. *Am J Respir Crit Care Med* 149: 825-833.

11. American Thoracic Society. 1999. Pulmonary rehabilitation. *Am J Respir Crit Care Med* 159: 1666-1682.

12. Hilling, L., and Smith, J. 1995. Pulmonary rehabilitation. In *Cardiopulmonary physical therapy,* 3rd ed. Edited by S. Irwin and J.S. Tecklin, 445-470. St. Louis: Mosby.

13. Chronic Obstructive Pulmonary Disease Surveillance—U.S. 1971-2000. *MMWR Morbidity and Mortality Weekly Report Surveillance Summaries* 51: SS-6.

14. Global Initiative for Chronic Obstructive Lung Disease. Available at: www.GOLDCOPD.com. Accessed September 2003.

15. American Lung Association. Estimated prevalence and incidence of lung disease by lung association territory. Available at: www.lungusa.org/data/ep/estimatedprev03.pdf. Accessed September 2003.

16. Centers for Disease Control. Facts about asthma. Available at: www.cdc.gov/od/oc/media/fact/asthma.htm. Accessed August 8, 1997.

17. Livingston, J.L., and Gillespie, M. 1935. The value of breathing exercises in asthma. *Lancet* 2: 705.

18. Miller, W.F. 1954. A physiologic evaluation of the effects of diaphragm breathing training in patients with chronic pulmonary emphysema. *Am J Med* 17: 471.

19. Dayman, H.G. 1956. Management of dyspnea in emphysema. *N Y J Med* 56: 1585.

20. Barach, A.L. 1959. Ambulatory oxygen therapy: Oxygen inhalation at home and out of doors. *Dis Chest* 35: 229.

21. Miller, W.F. 1967. Rehabilitation of patients with chronic obstructive lung disease. *Med Clin North Am* 51: 349.

22. Celli, B.R. Rassulo, J., and Make, B. 1968. Dyssynchronous breathing associated with arm but not leg exercise in patient with COPD. *N Engl J Med* 314: 1485-1490.

23. Haas, A., and Cardon, H. 1969. Rehabilitation in chronic obstructive pulmonary disease: A five-year study of 252 male patients. *Med Clin North Am* 53: 593.

24. Petty, T.L., Nett, L.M., Finigan, M.M., et al. 1969. A comprehensive care program for chronic airway obstruction: Methods and preliminary evaluation of symptomatic and functional improvement. *Ann Intern Med* 70: 1109.

25. Petty, T.L. 1970. Ambulatory care for emphysema and chronic bronchitis. *Chest* 58: 441.

26. Kass, I., and Dyksterhuis, J.E. 1971. The Nebraska COPD Rehabilitation Project: A program to identify the factors involved in the rehabilitation of patients with chronic obstructive pulmonary disease: A multidisciplinary study of 140 patients. Omaha: University of Nebraska. Final report, Social and Rehabilitation Service, DHEW Project RD-2517.

27. Wasserman, K., and Whipp, B.J. 1973. Exercise physiology in health and disease. *Am Rev Respir Dis* 112: 219.

28. Hodgkin, J.E., Balchum, O.J., Kass, I., et al. 1975. Chronic obstructive airway disease: Current concepts in diagnosis and comprehensive care. *JAMA* 232: 1243.

29. Nocturnal Oxygen Therapy Trial Group. 1980. Continuous or nocturnal oxygen therapy in hypoxemic chronic obstructive pulmonary disease: A clinical trial. *Ann Intern Med* 93: 391.

30. Dudley, D.L., Glaser, E.M., Jorgenson, M.S.W., et al. 1980. Psychosocial concomitants to rehabilitation in chronic obstructive pulmonary disease. Part I-III. *Chest* 77: 413.

31. Bebout, D.E., Hodgkin, J.E., Zorn, E.G., et al. 1983. Clinical and physiological outcomes of a university-hospital pulmonary rehabilitation program. *Respir Care* 28: 1468.

32. Mahler, D.A., Weinberg, D.H., Wells, C.K., et al. 1984. The measurement of dyspnea: Contents, interobserver agreement and physiological correlates of two new clinical indexes. *Chest* 85: 751-758.

33. Guyatt, G.H., Berman, L.B., Townsend, M., et al. 1987. A measure of quality of life for clinical trials in chronic lung disease. *Thorax* 42 (10): 773.

34. Casaburi, R., Patessio, A., Ioli, F., Zanaboni, S., Donner, C. F., and Wasserman, K. 1991. Reductions in exercise lactic acidosis and ventilation as a result of exercise training in patients with obstructive lung disease. *Am Rev Respir Dis* 143: 9-18.

35. Reardon, J., Awad, E., Normandine, E., et al. 1994. The effect of comprehensive outpatient pulmonary rehabilitation on dyspnea. *Chest* 105: 1046.

36. Goldstein, R.S., et al. 1994. Randomized controlled trial of respiratory rehabilitation. *Lancet* 344: 1394-1397.

37. Ries, A.L., Kaplan, R.M., Limberg, T.M., and Prewitt, L.M. 1995. Effects of pulmonary rehabilitation on physiologic and psychosocial outcomes in patients with chronic obstructive pulmonary disease. *Ann Intern Med* 122: 823-832.

38. Lacasse, Y., Wong, E., Guyatt, G.H., King, D., Cook, D.J., and Goldstein, R.S. 1996. Meta-analysis of respiratory rehabilitation in chronic obstructive pulmonary disease. *Lancet* 348: 1115-1119.

39. Maltais, F., LeBlanc, P., Simard, C., Jobin, J., Berube, C., Bruneau, J., Carrier, L., and Belleau, R. 1996. Skeletal muscle adaptation to endurance training in patients with chronic obstructive pulmonary disease. *Am J Respir Crit Care Med* 154: 442-447.

40. Griffiths, T.L., Burr, M.L., Campbell, I.A., Lewis-Jenkins, V., Mullins, J., Shiels, K., Turner-Lawlor, P.J., Payne, N., Newcombe, R.G., Lonescu, A.A., et al. 2000. Results at 1 year of outpatient multidisciplinary pulmonary rehabilitation: A randomized controlled trial. *Lancet* 355: 362-368.

41. Bourbeau, J., Julien, M., Maltais, F., Rouleau, M., Beaupre, A., Begin, R., Renzi, P., Nault, D., Borycki, E., Schwartzman, K., Singh, R., and Collet, J.P. 2003. Reduction in hospital utilization in patients with chronic obstructive pulmonary disease. *Arch Intern Med* 163: 585-591.

42. National Emphysema Treatment Trial Research Group. 2003. A randomized trial comparing lung-volume reduction surgery with medical therapy for severe emphysema. *N Engl J Med* 348: 2059.

43. Smoking and health: A report of the Advisory Committee to the Surgeon General. 1964. U.S. Department of Health, Education, and Welfare. PHS Publication 1103.

44. Office on Smoking and Health, ed. 1988. The health consequences of smoking: Nicotine addiction: A report of the Surgeon General. Washington, DC: U.S. Department of Health and Human Services, DHHS Publication CDC 88-8406.

45. Ries, A.L. 1990. Position paper of the American Association of Cardiovascular and Pulmonary Rehabilitation: Scientific basis of pulmonary rehabilitation. *J Cardiopulmon Rehabil* 10: 418.

46. American Association of Cardiovascular and Pulmonary Rehabilitation. 1993. *Guidelines for pulmonary rehabilitation programs*. Champaign, IL: Human Kinetics.

47. Fishman, A.P. 1994. Pulmonary rehabilitation research NIH workshop summary. *Am J Respir Crit Care Med* 149: 825.

48. American Thoracic Society. 1995. Standards for the diagnosis and care of patients with chronic obstructive pulmonary disease (COPD) and asthma. *Am Rev Respir Dis* 152: S78-S121.

49. European Respiratory Task Force. 1997. Position paper: Selection criteria and programs for pulmonary rehabilitation in COPD patients. *Eur Respir J* 10: 744.

50. National Lung Health Education Program (NLHEP) Executive Committee. 1998. Strategies in preserving lung health and preventing COPD and associated diseases. *Chest* 113 (2 Suppl).

51. American Thoracic Society. 1999. Dyspnea: Mechanisms, assessment and management: A consensus statement. *Am J Respir Crit Care Med* 159 (1): 321-340.

52. Hodgkin, J.E., Hilling, L., et al. 2002. American Association of Respiratory Care clinical practice guidelines: Pulmonary rehabilitation. *Respir Care* 47 (5): 617.

53. British Thoracic Society Standards of Care Subcommittee on Pulmonary Rehabilitation. 2001. Pulmonary rehabilitation. *Thorax* 5 (11): 827-834.

54. Hodgkin, J.E., Celli, B.R., and Connors, G.L., eds. 2000. *Pulmonary rehabilitation: Guidelines to success*, 3rd ed. Philadelphia: Lippincott Williams & Wilkins.

55. Casaburi, R., and Petty, T.L. l993. *Principles and practice of pulmonary rehabilitation.* Philadelphia: Saunders.

56. Jobin, J., Maltais, F., Poirier, P., et al., eds. 2002. *Advancing the frontiers of cardiopulmonary rehabilitation.* Champaign, IL: Human Kinetics.

57. Carlin, B.W., and Lingat, M. 2000. Preventive aspects for the patient with chronic lung disease. In *Pulmonary rehabilitation: Guidelines to success*, 3rd ed. Edited by J.E. Hodgkin, B.R. Celli, and G.L. Connors, 335. Philadelphia: Lippincott Williams & Wilkins.

58. Tiep, B.L. 1997. Disease management of COPD with pulmonary rehabilitation. *Chest* 112 (6): 1630-1656.

59. Centers for Disease Control. Smoking among U.S. adults. Fact sheets. Available at: www.cdc/gpv/od/oc/media/fact/smok1995.htm. Accessed December 24, 1997.

60. Centers for Disease Control. Tobacco use among middle and high school students. Available at: www.cdc.gov/tobacco/research_data/youth/mmwr5245_intro.htm. Accessed June 7, 2004.

Chapter 2

1. American Thoracic Society. 1999. Dyspnea. Mechanisms, assessment, and management: A consensus statement. *Am J Respir Crit Care Med* 159 (1): 321-340.

2. Mahler, D.A., and Jones, P.W. 1997. Measurement of dyspnea and quality of life in advanced lung disease. *Clin Chest Med* 18 (3): 457-469.

3. ZuWallack, R.L. 1998. Selection criteria and outcome assessment in pulmonary rehabilitation. *Monaldi Archives for Chest Dis* 53 (4): 429-437.

4. Resnikoff, P.M., and Ries, A.L. 1998. Pulmonary rehabilitation for chronic lung disease. *J Heart & Lung Transplant* 17 (7): 643-650.

5. American Thoracic Society. 1999. Pulmonary rehabilitation. *Am J Respir Crit Care Med* 159 (5 Pt. 1): 1666-1682.

6. Pierson, D.J., and Wilkins, R.L. 1992. Clinical skills in respiratory care. In *Foundations of respiratory care,* edited by D.J. Pierson and R.M. Kacmarek, 431-445. New York: Churchill Livingstone.

7. Connors, G.L., Hilling, L.R., and Morris, K.V. 1993. Assessment of the pulmonary rehabilitation candidate. In *Pulmonary rehabilitation: Guidelines to success*, 2nd ed. Edited by J.E. Hodgkin, G.L. Connors, and C.W. Bell, 64-68. Philadelphia: Lippincott Williams & Wilkins.

8. Gosselink, R., Troosters, T., and Decramer, M. 1997. Exercise training in COPD patients: The basic questions. *Eur Respir J* 10 (12): 2884-2891.

9. Casaburi, R. 2000. Skeletal muscle function in COPD. *Chest* 117 (5 Suppl. 1): 267S-271S.

10. Reed, K.L. 1991. Cardiopulmonary disorders. In *Quick reference to occupational therapy,* 195-209. Gaithersburg, MD: Aspen.

11. Selecky, P.A. 1993. Sexuality and the patient with lung disease. In *Principles and practice of pulmonary rehabilitation,* edited by R. Casaburi and T.L. Petty, 382-391. Philadelphia: Saunders.

12. Schols, A.M., and Wouters, E.F. 2000. Nutritional abnormalities and supplementation in chronic obstructive pulmonary disease. *Clinics in Chest Medicine* 21 (4): 753-762.

13. Wouters, E.F. 2000. Nutrition and metabolism in COPD. *Chest* 117 (5 Suppl. 1): 274S-280S.

14. Schols, A.M. 2000. Nutrition in chronic obstructive pulmonary disease. *Curr Opin Pulm Dis* 6 (2): 110-115.

15. Chapman, K.M., and Winter, W. 1996. COPD: Using nutrition to prevent respiratory function decline. *Geriatrics* 51 (12): 37-42.

16. Gilmartin, M.E. 1986. Patient and family education. *Clin Chest Med* 7 (4): 619-627.

Chapter 3

1. American Thoracic Society. 1999. ATS statement: Pulmonary rehabilitation—1999. *Am J Respir Crit Care Med* 159: 1673.

2. Scherer, Y.K., Schmieder, L.E., and Shimmel, S. 1998. The effects of education alone and in combination with pulmonary rehabilitation on self-efficacy in patients with COPD. *Rehabil Nurs* 23 (2): 71-77.

3. Lareau, S.C., and Insel, K.C. 2000. Education of patient and family. In *Pulmonary rehabilitation: Guidelines to success*, 3rd ed. Edited by J.E. Hodgkin, B.R. Celli, and G.L. Connors, 72-85. Philadelphia: Lippincott Williams & Wilkins.

4. Make, B. 1994. Collaborative self-management strategies for patients with respiratory disease. *Respir Care* 39: 566-579.

5. Mast, M.E., and VanAtta, M.J. 1986. Applying adult learning principles in instructional module design. *Nurse Educ* 11 (1): 35.

6. Babcock, D.E., and Miller, M.A. 1994. The adult learner. In *Client education: Theory and practice,* 19-25. St. Louis: Mosby.

7. American College of Chest Physicians. 1996. Clinical practice guideline: Providing patient and caregiver training. *Respir Care* 41 (7): 658-663.

8. Owen, P., Johnson, E., Frost, C., Porter, K., and O'Hare, E. 1993. Reading, readability, and patient education materials. *Cardiovasc Nurs* 29: 9-13.

9. Lipson, J., Dibble, S., and Minarik, P. 1996. *Culture and nursing care: A pocket guide.* San Francisco: UCSF Nursing Press.

10. American College of Chest Physicians and American Association of Cardiovascular and Pulmonary Rehabilitation Guidelines Panel. 1997. Pulmonary rehabilitation: Joint ACCP/AACVPR evidence-based guidelines. *Chest* 112 (5): 1363-1396.

11. West, J. 2001. *Pulmonary physiology and pathophysiology: An integrated, case-based approach.* Philadelphia: Lippincott Williams & Wilkins.

12. Ries, A.L., Bullock, P.J., Larsen, C.A., Limberg, T.M., Myers, R., Pfister, T., Sassi-Dambron, D.E., and Shelton, J.B. 2001. *Shortness of breath: A guide to better living and breathing,* 6th ed. St Louis: Mosby.

13. Morris, K., and Hodgkin, J. 1996. *Pulmonary rehabilitation administration and patient education manual.* Gaithersburg, MD: Aspen.

14. Pierson, D.J., and Kacmarek, R.M., eds. 1992. *Foundations of respiratory care.* New York: Churchill Livingstone.

15. National Heart, Lung and Blood Institute. 1997. *Expert panel report 2: Guidelines for the diagnosis and management of asthma.* NIH Publication No. 97-4051. Bethesda, MD: Author.

16. National Heart, Lung and Blood Institute. 1993. *Chronic obstructive pulmonary disease.* NIH Publication No. 93-2020. Bethesda, MD: Author.

17. Parsons, P., and Heffner, J.E., eds. 2002. *Pulmonary/respiratory therapy secrets,* 2nd ed. Philadelphia: Hanley & Belfus.

18. Steele, B. 1996. Timed walking tests of exercise capacity in chronic cardiopulmonary illness. *J Cardiopulm Rehabil* 16: 25-33.

19. Enright, P.L., and Hodgkin, J.E. 1997. Pulmonary function tests. In *Respiratory care: A guide to clinical practice,* edited by G.G. Burton, J.E. Hodgkin, and J.J. Ward, 225-248. Philadelphia: Lippincott.

20. Wasserman, K., Hansen, J., Sue, D., and Casaburi, R. 1999. *Principles of exercise testing and interpretation,* 3rd ed. Philadelphia: Lippincott Williams & Wilkins.

21. Kacmarek, R. 1992. Assessment of gas exchange and acid-base balance. In *Foundations of respiratory care,* edited by D.J. Pierson and R.M. Kacmarek, 477-512. New York: Churchill Livingstone.

22. Sinex, J.E. 1999. Pulse oximetry: Principles and limitations. *Am J Emerg Med* 17 (1): 59-67.

23. American College of Chest Physicians. 1991. Clinical practice guideline: Pulse oximetry. *Respir Care* 36 (12): 1406-1409.

24. Faling, L.J. 1993. Controlled breathing techniques and chest physical therapy in chronic obstructive pulmonary disease and allied conditions. In *Principles and practice of pulmonary rehabilitation,* edited by R. Casaburi and T.L. Petty, 167-174. Philadelphia: Saunders.

25. Hilling, L., and Smith, J. 1995. Pulmonary rehabilitation. In *Cardiopulmonary physical therapy,* 3rd ed. Edited by S. Irwin and J.S. Tecklin, 458-459. St Louis: Mosby.

26. Ries, A.L., Bullock, P.J., Larsen, C.A., Limberg, T.M., Myers, R., Pfister, T., Sassi-Dambron, D.E., and Shelton, J.B. 2001. *Shortness of breath: A guide to better living and breathing,* 6th ed. St Louis: Mosby.

27. Hillegass, E.H., and Sadowsky, H.S., eds. 2001. *Essentials of cardiopulmonary physical therapy,* 2nd ed. Philadelphia: Saunders.

28. Tiep, B., et al. 1986. Pursed-lip breathing training using ear oximetry. *Chest* 90: 218-221.

29. Hess, D.R. 2001. The evidence for secretion clearance techniques. *Respir Care* 46 (11): 1276-1292.

30. American College of Chest Physicians. 1993. Clinical practice guideline: Directed cough. *Respir Care* 38 (5): 495-499.

31. American College of Chest Physicians. 1991. Clinical practice guideline: Postural drainage therapy. *Respir Care* 36 (12): 1418-1426.

32. American College of Chest Physicians. 1993. Clinical practice guideline: Use of positive airway pressure adjuncts to bronchial hygiene therapy. *Respir Care* 38 (5): 516-521.

33. Fink, J.B. 2002. Positive pressure techniques for airway clearance. *Respir Care* 47 (7): 786-796.

34. Lapin, C.D. 2002. Airway physiology, autogenic drainage, and active cycle of breathing. *Respir Care* 47 (7): 778-785.

35. Weg, J.G. 1997. Bronchodilators in lung disease. In *Pulmonary disease diagnosis and therapy,* eds. M.G. Kahn and J.P. Lynch III, 143-75. Philadelphia: Lippincott Williams & Wilkins.

36. Cooper, C.B. 1993. Long-term oxygen therapy. In *Principles and practice of pulmonary rehabilitation,* eds. R. Casaburi and T.L. Petty, 183-203. Philadelphia: Saunders.

37. Nocturnal Oxygen Trial Group. 1980. Continuous or nocturnal oxygen therapy in hypoxemic chronic lung disease: A clinical trial. *Ann Intern Med* 93: 391-398.

38. American College of Chest Physicians and American Association of Cardiovascular and Pulmonary Rehabilitation Guidelines Panel. 1997. Pulmonary rehabilitation: Joint ACCP/AACVPR evidence-based guidelines. *Chest* 112 (5): 1365-1371.

39. Casaburi, R. 1993. Exercise training in chronic obstructive lung disease. In *Principles and practice of pulmonary rehabilitation,* eds. R. Casaburi and T.L. Petty, 204-224. Philadelphia: Saunders.

40. Rashbaum, I., and Whyte, N. 1996. Occupational therapy in pulmonary rehabilitation: Energy conservation and work simplification techniques. *Phys Med Rehabil Clin N Am* 7: 325.

41. Burns, M.R. 2000. Social and recreational support for the pulmonary patient. In *Pulmonary rehabilitation: Guidelines to success,* 3rd ed. Edited by J.E. Hodgkin, B.R. Celli, and G.L. Connors, 465-477. Philadelphia: Lippincott Williams & Wilkins.

42. Selecky, P.A. 2000. Sexuality in the pulmonary patient. In *Pulmonary rehabilitation: Guidelines to success,* 3rd ed. Edited by J.E. Hodgkin, B.R. Celli, and G.L. Connors, 317-334. Philadelphia: Lippincott Williams & Wilkins.

43. Stoller, J.K. 2000. Oxygen and air travel. *Respir Care* 45 (2): 214-221.

44. Fink, J.B. 2000. Metered-dose inhalers, dry powder inhalers, and transitions. *Respir Care* 45 (6): 623-635.

45. American College of Chest Physicians. 1992. Clinical practice guideline: Selection of aerosol delivery device. *Respir Care* 37 (8): 891-897.

46. National Heart, Lung and Blood Institute. 1997. *Expert panel report 2: Practical guide for the diagnosis and management of asthma.* NIH Publication No. 97-4057, 48-9. Bethesda, MD: Author.

47. Kacmarek, R.M. 2000. Delivery systems for long-term oxygen. *Respir Care* 45 (1): 84-92.

48. McCoy, R. 2000. Oxygen-conserving techniques and devices. *Respir Care* 45 (1): 95-103.

49. Hoffman, L.A. 1994. Novel strategies for delivering oxygen: Reservoir cannula, demand flow, and transtracheal oxygen administration. *Respir Care* 39 (4): 363-377.

50. Covey, M.K, Larson, J.L., Wirtz, S.E., Berry, J.K., Pogue, N.J., Alex, C.G., and Patel, M. 2001. High-intensity inspiratory muscle training in patients with chronic obstructive pulmonary disease and severely reduced function. *J Cardiopulm Rehabil* 21 (4): 231-240.

51. American College of Chest Physicians. 1999. Suctioning of the patient in the home. *Respir Care* 44 (1): 99-104.

52. Tamburri, L.M. 2000. Care of the patient with a tracheostomy. *Orthop Nurs* 19 (2): 49-58.

53. American College of Chest Physicians. 1995. Clinical practice guideline: Long-term invasive mechanical ventilation in the home. *Respir Care* 40 (12): 1313-1320.

54. Goldberg, A.I. 2002. Noninvasive mechanical ventilation at home: Building on tradition. *Chest* 121 (2): 415-421.

55. Fiore, M.C. 2000. U.S. public health service clinical practice guideline: Treating tobacco use and dependence. *Respir Care* 45 (10): 1200-1262.

56. Berry, J.K., and Baum, C.L. 2001. Malnutrition in chronic obstructive pulmonary disease: Adding insult to injury. *AACN Clin Issues* 12 (2): 210-219.

57. Foley, R.J., and ZuWallack, R. 2001. The impact of nutritional depletion in chronic obstructive pulmonary disease. *J Cardiopulm Rehabil* 21 (5): 288-295.

58. Slinde, F., Gronberg, A.M., Engstrom, C.R., Rossander-Hulthen, L., and Larsson, S. 2002. Individual dietary intervention in patients with COPD during multidisciplinary rehabilitation. *Respir Med* 96 (5): 330-336.

59. Heffner, J.E., Fahy, B., and Barbieri, C. 1996. Advance directive education during pulmonary rehabilitation. *Chest* 109: 373-379.

60. Heffner, J.E., et al. 1996. Attitudes regarding advance directives among patients in pulmonary rehabilitation. *Am J Respir Crit Care Med* 154: 1735-1740.

61. Heffner, J.E., et al. 1997. Outcomes of advance directive education of pulmonary rehabilitation patients. *Am J Respir Crit Care Med* 155: 1055-1059.

62. Petty, T.L., and Nett, L.M. 2002. *Enjoying life with chronic obstructive pulmonary disease,* 3rd ed. Cedar Grove, NJ: Laennec.

Chapter 4

1. American College of Chest Physicians and American Association for Cardiovascular and Pulmonary Rehabilitation. 1997. Pulmonary rehabilitation. Joint ACCP/AACVPR evidence-based guidelines. *Chest* 112 (5): 1363-1396.

2. Wasserman, K., et al. 1994. *Principles of exercise testing and interpretation.* Philadelphia: Lea & Febiger.

3. ACSM. 1995. *American College of Sports Medicine's guidelines for exercise testing and prescription,* 5th ed. Baltimore, MD: Williams & Wilkins.

4. Ries, A.L. 1994. The importance of exercise in pulmonary rehabilitation. *Clin Chest Med* 15 (2): 327-337.

5. Belman, M.J. Exercise in patients with chronic obstructive pulmonary disease. *Thorax* 48 (9): 936-946.

6. Casaburi, R., Patessio, A., Ioli, F., et al. 1991. Reductions in exercise lactic acidosis and ventilation as a result of exercise training in patients with obstructive lung disease. *Am Rev Respir Dis* 143: 9-18.

7. Ries, A.L., Farrow, J.T., and Clausen, J.L. 1988. Pulmonary function tests cannot predict exercise-induced hypoxemia in chronic obstructive pulmonary disease. *Chest* 93 (3): 454-459.

8. American Thoracic Society Committee on Pulmonary Function Standards. 2000. Guidelines for methacholine and exercise challenge testing —1999. *Am J of Resp & Crit Care Med* 161: 309-329.

9. ATS Committee on Proficiency Standards for Clinical Pulmonary Function Laboratories. 2002. ATS statement: Guidelines for the six-minute walk test. *Am J of Resp & Crit Care Med* 166: 111-117.

10. Steele, B. 1996. Time walking tests of exercise capacity in chronic cardiopulmonary illness. *J Cardiopulm Rehabil* 16: 25.

11. Morales, F.J., Montemayor, T., and Martinez, A. 2000. Shuttle vs. 6-minute walk test in the prediction of outcome in chronic heart failure. *Int J Cardiol* 76: 101-105.

12. Revill, S.M., Morgan, M.D.L., Singh, S.J., et al. 1999. The endurance shuttle walk: A new field test for the assessment of endurance capacity in COPD. *Thorax* 54: 213-222.

13. Singh, S.J., Morgan, M.D., Hardman, A.E. 1994. Comparison of oxygen uptake during a conventional treadmill test and the shuttle walk test in chronic airflow limitation, *Eur Respir J* 7: 2016-2020.

14. Johnson, B.D., Weisman, I.M., Zeballos, R.J., and Beck, K.C. 1999. Emerging concepts in the evaluation of ventilatory limitation during exercise: The exercise tidal flow-volume loop. *Chest* 116 (2): 488-503.

15. Borg, G.A. 1998. *Borg's perceived exertion and pain scales.* Champaign: Human Kinetics.

16. Home, D., and Corsello, P. 1993. Physical and occupational therapy for patients with chronic lung disease. *Sem Respir Med* 14 (6): 466-481.

17. Hillegass, E.A., and Sadowsky, H.S. 1994. *Essentials of cardiopulmonary physical therapy.* Philadelphia: W.B. Saunders.

18. Gallagher, C.G. 1994. Exercise limitation and clinical exercise testing in chronic obstructive pulmonary disease. *Clin Chest Med* 15: 305-326.

19. Richardson, R.S., Sheldon, J., Poole, D.C., Hopkins, S.R., Ries, A.L., and Wagner, P.D. 1999. Evidence of skeletal muscle metabolic reserve during whole body exercise in patients with chronic obstructive pulmonary disease. *Am J Respir Crit Care Med* 159: 881-885.

20. Nici, L. 2000. Mechanisms and measures of exercise intolerance in chronic obstructive pulmonary disease. *Clin Chest Med* 21 (4): 693-704.

21. Haccoun, C., Smountas, A.A., Gibbons, W.J., Bourbeau, J., and Lands, L.C. 2002. Isokinetic muscle function in COPD. *Chest* 121: 1079-1084.

22. O'Donnell, D.E. 2001. Ventilatory limitations in chronic obstructive pulmonary disease. *Med Sci Sports Exerc* 33 (7 Suppl): S647-S655.

23. Fitting, J.W. 2001. Respiratory muscles in chronic obstructive pulmonary disease. *Swiss Med Weekly* 131: 483-486.

24. Sietsema, K. 2001. Cardiovascular limitations in chronic obstructive pulmonary disease. *Med Sci Sports Exerc* 33 (7 Suppl): S656-S661.

25. Killian, K.J., LeBlanc, P., Martin, D.H., et al. 1992. Exercise capacity and ventilatory, circulatory and symptom limitation in patients with chronic airflow obstruction. *Am Rev Respir Dis* 146: 935-940.

26. Casaburi, R. 2001. Skeletal muscle dysfunction in chronic obstructive pulmonary disease. *Med Sci Sports Exerc* 33 (7 Suppl): S662-S670.

27. American Thoracic Society/European Respiratory Society. 1999. Skeletal muscle dysfunction in chronic obstructive pulmonary disease. *Am J Respir Crit Care Med* 159: S1-S40.

28. Baarends, E.M., Schols, A.M.W.J., Mostert, R., and Wouters, E.F.M. 1997. Peak exercise response in relation to tissue depletion in patients with chronic obstructive pulmonary disease. *Eur Respir J* 10: 2807-2813.

29. Bernard, S., LeBlanc, P., Whittom, F., et al. 1998. Peripheral muscle weakness in patients with chronic obstructive pulmonary disease. *Am J Respir Crit Care Med* 158: 629-634.

30. Hilderbrand, I.L., Sylven, C., Esbjonrsson, M., Hellstrom, K., and Jansson, E. 1991. Does chronic hypoxemia induce transformation of fiber types? *Acta Physiol Scand* 141: 435-439.

31. Jakobsson, P., Jordfelt, I., and Brundin, A. 1990. Skeletal muscle metabolites and fiber types in patients with advanced COPD with and without chronic respiratory failure. *Eur Respir J* 3: 192-196.

32. Hughes, R.L., Katz, H., Sahgal, J.A., Campbell, J.A., Hartz, R., and Shields, T.Q. 1983. Fiber size and energy metabolites in 5 separate muscles from patients with chronic obstructive lung disease. *Respiration* 44: 321-328.

33. Simard, C., Maltais, F., LeBlanc, P., et al. 1996. Mitochondrial and capillarity changes in the vastus lateralis muscle of COPD patients: Electron microscopy study. *Med Sci Sports Exerc* 28: S95.

34. Jakobsson, P., Jordfelt, I., and Henriksson, J. 1995. Metabolic enzyme activity in the quadriceps femoris muscle in patients with severe COPD. *Am J Respir Crit Care Med* 151: 374-377.

35. Maltais, F., Simard, A.A., Simard, C., et al. 1996. Oxidative capacity of the skeletal muscle and lactic acid kinetics during exercise in normal subjects and in patients with COPD. *Am J Respir Crit Care Med* 153: 288-293.

36. Gosker, H.R., van Mameren, H., Dijk, P.J., Engelen, M.P.K.J., van der Vusse, G.J., Wouters, E.F.M., and Schols, A.M.W.J. 2002. Skeletal muscle fiber type-shifting and metabolic profile in patients with chronic obstructive pulmonary disease. *Eur Respir J* 19: 617-625.

37. Mador, M.J., Kufel, T.J., and Pineda, L. 2000. Quadriceps fatigue after cycle exercise in patients with chronic obstructive pulmonary disease. *Am J Respir Crit Care Med* 161: 447-453.

38. Serres, I., Gautier, V., Varray, A., and Prefaut, C. 1998. Impaired skeletal muscle endurance related to physical inactivity and altered lung function in COPD patients. *Chest* 113: 900-905.

39. Maltais, F., Jobin, J., Sullivan, M.J., Bernard, S., Whittom, F., Killian, K., et al. 1998. Metabolic and hemodynamic responses of lower limb during exercise in patients with COPD. *J Appl Physiol* 84 (5): 1573-1580.

40. Engelen, M.P., Schols, A.M., Does, J.D., Gosker, H.R., Deutz, N.E., and Wouters, E.F. 2000. Exercise-induced lactate increase in relation to muscle substrates in patients with chronic obstructive pulmonary disease. *Am J Respir Crit Care Med* 162 (5): 1697-1704.

41. Gosselink, R., Troosters, T., and Decramer, M. 1996. Peripheral muscle weakness contributes to exercise limitation in COPD. *Am J Respir Crit Care Med* 153: 976-980.

42. Hamilton, A.L., Killian, K.J., Summers, E., and Jones, N.L. 1995. Muscle strength, symptom intensity, and exercise capacity in patients with cardiorespiratory disorders. *Am J Respir Crit Care Med* 152: 2021-2031.

43. Polkey, M.I. 2002. Muscle metabolism and exercise tolerance in COPD. *Chest* 121: 131S-135S.

44. Debigare, R., Cote, C.H., and Maltais, F. 2001. Peripheral muscle wasting in chronic obstructive pulmonary disease. *Am J Respir Crit Care Med* 164: 1712-1717.

45. Wouters, E.F.M., Creutzberg, E.C., and Schols, A.M.W.J. 2002. Systemic effects in COPD. *Chest* 121 Suppl: 127S-130S.

46. Prefaut, C., Varray, A., and Vallet, G. 1995. Pathophysiological basis of exercise training in patients with chronic obstructive lung disease. *Eur Respir Rev* 5: 25, 27-32.

47. Plankeel, J., and MacIntyre, N.R. 2002. Mechanism of limitation predicts rehabilitation outcome in COPD. *Am J Resp Crit Care Med* 165: A156.

48. Casaburi, R., and Petty, T.L., eds. 1993. *Principles and practice of pulmonary rehabilitation.* Philadelphia: W.B. Saunders.

49. American Thoracic Society statement. 1999. Pulmonary rehabilitation—1999. *Am J Respir Crit Care Med* 159: 1666-1682.

50. Goldstein, R.S., Gort, E.H., Stubbing, D., Avendano, M.S., and Guyatt, G.H. 1994. Randomized controlled trial of respiratory rehabilitation. *Lancet* 344: 1394-1397.

51. Lacasse, Y., Wang, E., Guyatt, G., et al. 1996. Meta-analysis of respiratory rehabilitation in chronic obstructive pulmonary disease. *Lancet* 348: 1115-1119.

52. Goldstein, R.S., et al. 1994. Randomized controlled trial of respiratory rehabilitation. *Lancet* 1394-1397.

53. Ries, A.L., Kaplan, R.M., Limberg, T.M., and Prewitt, L. 1995. Effects of pulmonary rehabilitation on physiologic and psychological outcomes in patients with chronic obstructive pulmonary disease. *Ann Intern Med* 122: 823-832.

54. Reardon, J., et al. 1994. The effect of comprehensive outpatient pulmonary rehabilitation on dyspnea. *Chest* 105: 1046-1052.

55. Vale, F., Reardon, J.Z., and ZuWallack, R.L. 1993. The long-term benefits of outpatient pulmonary rehabilitation on exercise endurance and quality of life. *Chest* 103: 42-45.

56. Vogziatzis, I., Williamson, A.F., Miles, J., et al. 1999. Physiological response to moderate exercise workloads in a pulmonary rehabilitation program in patients with varying degrees of airflow obstruction. *Chest* 116: 1200-1207.

57. Maltais, F., LeBlanc, P., Simard, C., et al. 1996. Skeletal muscle adaptation to endurance training in patients with chronic obstructive pulmonary disease. *Am J Respir Crit Care Med* 154: 442-447.

58. Vallet, G., Ahmaidi, S., Serres, I., et al. 1997. Comparison of two training programmes in chronic airway limitation patients: Standardized versus individualized protocols. *Eur Respir J* 10: 114-122.

59. Gimenez, M., Servera, E., Vergara, P., Bach, J.R., and Polu, J.M. 2000. Endurance training in patients with chronic obstructive pulmonary disease: A comparison of high versus moderate intensity. *Arch Phys Med Rehabil* 81: 102-109.

60. Puente-Maestu, L., Sanz, M.L., Sanz, P., Ruiz de Ona, J.M., Rodriguez-Hermosa, J.L., and Whipp, B.J. 2000. Effects of two types of training on pulmonary and cardiac responses to moderate exercise in patients with COPD. *Eur Respir J* 15: 1026-1032.

61. Casaburi, R., Porszasz, J., Burns, M.R., et al. 1997. Physiologic benefits of exercise training in rehabilitation of patients with severe chronic obstructive pulmonary disease. *Am J Respir Crit Care Med* 155: 1541-1551.

62. Maltais, F., LeBlanc, P., Jobin, J., et al. 1997. Intensity of training and physiologic adaptation in patients with chronic obstructive pulmonary disease. *Am J Respir Crit Care Med* 155: 555-561.

63. Vogiatzis, I., Nanas, S., and Roussos, C. 2002. Interval training as an alternative modality to continuous exercise in patients with COPD. *Eur Respir J* 20: 12-19.

64. Coppoolse, R., Schols, A.M.W.J., Baarends, E.M., Mostert, R., Akkermans, M.A., Janssen, P.P., and Wouters, E.F.M. 1999. Interval versus continuous training in patients with severe COPD: A randomized clinical trial. *Eur Respir J* 14: 258-263.

65. Votto, J., Bowen, J., Scalise, P., Wollschlager, C., and ZuWallack, R. 1996. Short-stay comprehensive inpatient pulmonary rehabilitation for advanced chronic obstructive pulmonary disease. *Arch Phys Med Rehabil* 77: 1115-1118.

66. Clark, C.J., Cochrane, L., and Mackay, E. 1996. Low intensity peripheral muscle conditioning improves exercise tolerance and breathlessness in COPD. *Eur Respir J* 9: 2590-2596.

67. Normandin, E.A., McCusker, C., Connors, M.L., Vale, F., Gerardi, D., and ZuWallack, R.L. 2002. An evaluation of two approaches to exercise conditioning in pulmonary rehabilitation. *Chest* 121: 1085-1091.

68. Neder, J.A., Sword, D., Ward, S.A., Mackay, E., Cochrane, L.M., and Clark, C.J. 2002. Home-based neuromuscular electrical stimulation as a new rehabilitative strategy for severely disabled patients with chronic obstructive pulmonary disease (COPD). *Thorax* 57: 333-337.

69. Bourjeily-Habr, G., Rochester, C.L., Palermo, F., Snyder, P., and Mohsenin, V. 2002. Randomized controlled trial of transcutaneous electrical muscle stimulation of the lower extremities in patients with chronic obstructive pulmonary disease. *Thorax* 57: 1045-1049.

70. Nocturnal Oxygen Therapy Trial Group. 1980. Continuous or nocturnal oxygen therapy in hypoxemic chronic obstructive lung disease: A clinical trial. *Ann Intern Med* 93: 391-398.

71. American Thoracic Society. 1995. Standards for the diagnosis and care of patients with chronic obstructive pulmonary disease (COPD). *Am J Respir Crit Care Med* 136: 225-244.

72. Emtner, M., Porszasz, J., Burns, M., et al. 2003. Benefits of supplemental oxygen in exercise training in non-hypoxemic COPD patients. *Am J Resp Crit Care Med* 168: 1034-1042.

73. O'Donnell, D.E., McGuire, M., Samis, L., and Webb, K.A. 1995. The impact of exercise reconditioning on breathlessness in severe chronic airflow limitation. *Am J Respir Crit Care Med* 152: 2005-2013.

74. Wedzicha, J.A., Bestall, J.C., Garrod, R., et al. 1998. Randomized controlled trial of pulmonary rehabilitation in severe chronic obstructive pulmonary disease patients, stratified with the MRC dyspnea scale. *Eur Respir J* 12: 363-369.

75. Cambach, W., Wagenaar, R.C., Koelman, T.W., et al. 1999. The long-term effects of pulmonary rehabilitation in patients with asthma and chronic obstructive pulmonary disease: A research synthesis. *Arch Phys Med Rehabil* 80: 103-111.

76. Troosters, T., Gosselink, R., and Decramer, M. 2000. Short- and long-term effects of outpatient rehabilitation in patients with chronic obstructive pulmonary disease: A randomized trial. *Am J Med* 109: 207-212.

77. O' Holle, R.H., Williams, D.V., Vandree, R.B., et al. 1988. Increased muscle efficiency and sustained benefits in an outpatient community hospital-based pulmonary rehabilitation program. *Chest* 94: 1161-1168.

78. Cambach, W., Chadwick-Stravr, R.V.M., Wagenaar, R.C., van Kiempera, A.R.J., and Kemper, H.C.G. 1997. The effects of a community-based pulmonary rehabilitation programme on exercise tolerance and quality of life: A randomized controlled trial. *Eur Respir J* 10: 104-113.

79. Guell, R., Casan, P., Belda, J., Sangenis, M., Morante, F., Guyatt, G.H., and Sanchis, J. 2000. Long-term effects of outpatient rehabilitation of COPD: A randomized trial. *Chest* 117: 976-983.

80. Baarends, E.M., Schols, A.M.W.J., Slebos, D.J., et al. 1995. Metabolic and ventilatory response pattern to arm elevation in patients with COPD and healthy age-matched subjects. *Eur Respir J* 8: 1345-1351.

81. Martinez, F.J., Couser, J.I., and Celli, B.R. 1991. Respiratory response to arm elevation in patients with severe airflow obstruction. *Am Rev Respir Dis* 143 (103): 476-480.

82. Tangri, S., and Wolf, C.R. 1973. The breathing pattern in chronic obstructive lung disease during the performance of some daily activities. *Chest* 63: 126-127.

83. Celli, B.R., Rassulo, J., and Make, B.J. 1986. Dyssynchronous breathing during arm but not leg exercise in patients with chronic airflow obstruction. *N Engl J Med* 314: 1485-1490.

84. Celli, B.R. 1994. The clinical use of upper extremity exercise. *Clin Chest Med* 15 (2): 339-349.

85. Criner, G.J., and Celli, B.R. 1988. Effects of unsupported arm exercise on ventilatory muscle recruitment in patients with severe chronic airflow obstruction. *Am Rev Respir Dis* 138: 856-886.

86. Gea, J.G., Pasto, M., Carmona, M.A., Orozco-Levi, M., Palomeque, J., and Broquetas, J. 2001. Metabolic characteristics of the deltoid muscle in patients with chronic obstructive pulmonary disease. *Eur Respir J* 17: 939-945.

87. Gosselink, R., Troosters, T., and Decramer, M. 2000. Distribution of muscle weakness in patients with stable chronic obstructive pulmonary disease. *J Cardiopulm Rehabil* 20: 353-360.

88. Ries, A.L., and Moser, K.M. 1986. Comparison of isocapneic hyperventilation and walking exercise training at home in pulmonary rehabilitation. *Chest* 90: 285-289.

89. Simpson, K., Killian, K., McCartney, N., et al. 1992. Randomized controlled trial of weightlifting exercise in patients with chronic airflow limitation. *Thorax* 47: 70-75.

90. Couser, J.I., Maertinez, F.J., and Celli, B.R. 1993. Pulmonary rehabilitation that includes arm exercise reduces metabolic and ventilatory requirements for single arm elevation. *Chest* 103: 37-41.

91. Martinez, F.J., Vogel, P.D., Dupont, D.N., et al. 1993. Supported arm exercise vs. unsupported arm exercise in the rehabilitation of patients with severe chronic airflow obstruction. *Chest* 103: 1397-1402.

92. Ries, A.L., Ellis, B., and Hawkins, R. 1988. Upper extremity exercise training in chronic obstructive pulmonary disease. *Chest* 93 (4): 688-692.

93. Simpson, K., Killian, K., McCartney, N., et al. 1992. Randomized controlled trial of weightlifting exercise in patients with chronic airflow limitation. *Thorax* 47: 70-75.

94. Clark, C.J., Cochrane, L.M., Mackay, E., and Paton, B. 2000. Skeletal muscle strength and endurance in patients with mild COPD and the effects of weight training. *Eur Respir J* 15: 92-97.

95. Storer, T.W. 2001. Exercise in chronic pulmonary disease: Resistance exercise prescription *Med Sci Sports Exerc* 33 (7 Suppl): S680-S686.

96. Spruit, M.A., Gosselink, R., Troosters, T., De Paepe, K., and Decramer, M. 2002. Resistance versus endurance training in patients with COPD and peripheral muscle weakness. *Eur Respir J* 19: 1072-1078.

97. Ortega, F., Toral, J., Cejudo, P., Villagomez, R., Sanchez, H., Castillo, J., and Montemayor, T. 2002. Comparison of effects of strength and endurance training in patients with chronic obstructive pulmonary disease. *Am J Respir Crit Care Med* 166: 669-674.

98. Bernard, S., Whittom, F., LeBlanc, P., et al. 1999. Aerobic and strength training in patients with chronic obstructive pulmonary disease. *Am J Respir Crit Care Med* 59: 896-901.

99. Alter, M.J. 1988. *Science of stretching.* Champaign, IL: Human Kinetics.

100. Harver, A., Mahler, D.A., and Daubenspeck, J.A. 1989. Targeted inspiratory muscle training improves respiratory muscle function and reduces dyspnea in patients with chronic obstructive pulmonary disease. *Ann Intern Med* 111: 117-124.

101. Patessio, A., et al. 1989. Relationship between perception of breathlessness and inspiratory resistive loading: Report on a clinical trial. *Eur Respir J* 2: 587-591 s.

102. Leith, D.E., and Bradley, M. 1976. Ventilatory muscle strength and endurance training. *J Appl Physiol* 41 (4): 508-516.

103. Belman, M.J., and Shadmehr, R. 1988. Targeted resistive ventilatory muscle training in chronic obstructive pulmonary disease. *J Appl Physiol* 65 (6): 2726-2735.

104. Goldstein, R.S. Ventilatory muscle training. *Thorax* 48: 1025-1033.

105. Smith, K., et al. 1992. Respiratory muscle training in chronic airflow limitation: A meta-analysis. *Am Rev Respir Dis* 145: 533-539.

106. Belman, M.J., et al. 1994. Ventilatory load characteristics during ventilatory muscle training. *Am J Respir Crit Care Med* 149: 925-929.

107. Wijkstra, P.J., van der Mark, T.W., Kraan, J., et al. 1996. Long-term effects of home rehabilitation on physical performance in chronic obstructive pulmonary disease. *Am J Respir Crit Care Med* 153: 1234-1241.

108. Wijkstra, P.J., van der Mark, T.W., Kraan, J., et al. 1996. Effects of home rehabilitation on physical performance in chronic obstructive pulmonary disease (COPD). *Eur Respir J* 9: 104-110.

Chapter 5

1. Dudley, D.L., Wermuth, C., and Hague, W. 1973. Psychosocial aspects of care in the chronic obstructive pulmonary disease patient. *Heart Lung* 2: 289.

2. Prigatano, G.P., Wright, E.C., and Levin, D. 1984. Quality of life and its predictors in patients with mild hypoxemia and chronic obstructive pulmonary disease. *Arch Intern Med* 144: 1613-1619.

3. Heim, E., Blaser, A., and Waidelich, E. 1972. Dyspnea: Psychophysiologic relationships. *Psychosom Med* 34: 405.

4. Toms, J., and Harrison, K. 2002. Living with chronic lung disease and the effect of pulmonary rehabilitation: Patients' perspectives. *Physiotherapy* 88 (10): 605-619.

5. Leidy, N.K., and Traver, G.A. 1996. Adjustment and social behavior in older adults with chronic obstructive pulmonary disease: The family's perspective. *J Adv Nurs* 23: 252-259.

6. Agle, D.P., and Baum, G.L. 1977. Psychological aspects of chronic obstructive pulmonary disease. *Med Clin North Am* 61: 749-758.

7. McSweeny, A.J., et al. 1982. Life quality of patients with chronic obstructive pulmonary disease. *Arch Intern Med* 142: 473-478.

8. van Ede, L., et al. 1999. Prevalence of depression in patients with chronic obstructive pulmonary disease: A systematic review. *Thorax* 54: 699-702.

9. American Psychiatric Association. 1994. *Diagnostic and statistical manual of mental disorders*, 4th ed. Washington, DC: American Psychiatric Association.

10. Dudley, D.L., Glaser, E.M., Jorgenson, B.N., and Logan, D.L. 1980. Psychosocial concomitants to rehabilitation in chronic obstructive pulmonary disease. *Chest* 77 (3): 413-420.

11. Farkas, S.W. 1980. Impact of chronic illness on the patient's spouse. *Health Soc Work* 5 (4): 39-46.

12. Kim, H.F.S., et al. 2000. Functional impairment in COPD patients: The impact of anxiety and depression. *Psychosomatics* 41: 465-471.

13. Ormel, J., et al. 1998. Functioning, well-being, and health perception in late middle-aged and older people: Comparing the effects of depressive symptoms and chronic medical conditions. *J Am Geriatr Soc* 46: 39-48.

14. Miller, W.R., and Rollnick, S. 1991. *Motivational interviewing: Preparing people to change addictive behavior*. New York: Guilford Press.

15. Becker, M.H., Maiman, L.A., Kirscht, J.P., Haefner, D.P., Drackman, R.H., and Taylor, D.W. 1979. Patient perceptions and compliance: Recent studies of the health belief model. In *Compliance in health care*, R.B. Haynes, D.W. Taylor, and D.L. Sackett, eds. 78-109. Baltimore: Johns Hopkins University Press.

16. Bandura, A. 1991. Self-efficacy mechanism in physiological activation and health-promoting behavior. *Adaptation, learning and affect*. J.I. Madden, S. Matthysse, and J. Barchas, eds. 229. New York: Raven Press.

17. Kohler, C.L., Fish, L., Greene, P.G. 2002. The relationship of perceived self-efficacy to quality of life in chronic obstructive pulmonary disease. *Health Psychology* 21 (6): 610-614.

18. Young, Y., et al. 1999. Predictors of non-adherence to a pulmonary rehabilitation program. *Eur Respir J* 13: 855-859.

19. Lacasse, Y., Wong, E., Guyatt, G.G., et al. 1996. Meta-analysis of respiratory rehabilitation in chronic obstructive pulmonary disease. *Lancet* 348: 1115-1119.

20. Prochaska, J.O., and Velicer, W.F. 1997. The transtheoretical model of health behavior change. *Am J Health Prom* 12: 38-48.

21. Prochaska, J.O., et al. 1988. Measuring processes of change: Applications to the cessation of smoking. *J Consult Clin Psychol* 56: 520-528.

22. Fiore, M.C., et al. 2000. Treating tobacco use and dependence. *Clinical practice guidelines*. Rockville, MD: U.S. Department of Health and Human Services.

23. Haynes, R.B. 1979. Determinants of compliance: The disease and mechanics of treatment. *Compliance in health care*. R.B. Haynes, D.W. Taylor, and D.L. Sackett, eds. 49-62. Baltimore: Johns Hopkins University Press.

24. Rand, C.S. 1998. Patient and regimen-related factors that influence compliance with asthma therapy. *Eur Respir Rev* 8 (56): 270-274.

25. Jones, P.W. 1998. Health status, quality of life and compliance. *Eur Respir Rev* 8 (56): 243-246.

26. Strauss, A.L., et al. 1984. *Chronic illness and the quality of life*. St. Louis: Mosby.

27. Ries, A.L. 1990. Position paper of the American Association of Cardiovascular and Pulmonary Rehabilitation: Scientific basis of pulmonary rehabilitation. *J Cardiopulm Rehabil* 10: 418-441.

28. McCathie, H.C.F., et al. 2002. Adjustment to chronic obstructive pulmonary disease: The importance of psychological factors. *Eur Respir J* 19: 47-53.

29. Crockett, A.J., Smith, B.J., Hender, K., et al. 2003. Systematic assessment of clinical practice guidelines for the management of chronic obstructive pulmonary disease. *Respiratory Medicine* 97 (1): 37-45.

30. Bergs, D. 2002. "The hidden client"—women caring for husbands with COPD: Their experience of quality of life. *J Clin Nurs* 11 (5): 613-621.

31. Cannon, C.A., and Cavanaugh, J.C. 1998. Chronic illness in the context of marriage: A systems perspective of stress and coping on chronic obstructive pulmonary disease. *Fam Sys Health* 6 (4): 401-418.

32. Sotile, W.M. 1996. *Psychosocial interventions for cardiopulmonary patients*. Champaign, IL: Human Kinetics.

33. Singer, H.K., Ruchinskas, R.A., Riley, K.C., et al. 2001. The psychological impact of end-stage lung disease. *Chest* 120 (4): 1246-1252.

34. Lacasse, Y., et al. 2001. Prevalence of depressive symptoms and depression in patients with severe oxygen-dependent chronic obstructive pulmonary disease. *J Cardiopulm Rehabil* 20: 80-86.

35. Mills, T.L. 2001. Comorbid depressive symptomatology: Isolating the effects of chronic medical conditions of self-reported depressive symptoms among community-dwelling older adults. *Social Science & Medicine* 53 (5): 569-578.

36. Yohannes, A.M., et al. 2000. Mood disorders in elderly patients with chronic obstructive pulmonary disease. *Rev Clin Gerontol* 10: 193-202.

37. Yohannes, A.M., Baldwin, R.C., and Connolly, M.J. 2003. Prevalence of sub-threshold depression in elderly patients with chronic obstructive pulmonary disease. *Int J Geriatr Psychiatry* 18 (5): 412-416.

38. Ibenz, M., Aguilar, J.J., Maderal, M.A., et al. 2001. Sexuality in chronic respiratory failure: Coincidences and divergences between patient and primary caregiver. *Respiratory Medicine* 95 (12): 975-979.

39. Schonhofer, B., von Sydow, K., Bucher, T., et al. 2001. Sexuality in patients with noninvasive mechanical ventilation due to chronic respiratory failure. *Am J Respir Crit Care Med* 164 (9): 1612-1617.

40. Emery, C.F. 1995. Adherence in cardiac and pulmonary rehabilitation. *J Cardiopulm Rehabil* 15: 420-423.

41. Emery, C.F., et al. 1994. Psychological functioning among middle-aged and older adult pulmonary patients in exercise rehabilitation. *Phys Occup Ther Geriatr* 12: 13-26.

42. Emery, C.F., et al. 1991. Psychological outcomes of a pulmonary rehabilitation program. *Chest* 100: 613-617.

43. Ries, A.L., et al. 1995. Effects of pulmonary rehabilitation on physiologic and psychosocial outcomes in patients with chronic obstructive pulmonary disease. *Ann Intern Med* 122: 823-832.

44. Emery, C.F., et al. 1998. Psychological and cognitive outcomes of a randomized trial of exercise among patients with chronic obstructive pulmonary disease. *Health Psychology* 17 (3): 232-240.

45. Kozora, E., Tran, Z.V., and Make, B. 2002. Neurobehavioral improvement after brief rehabilitation in patients with chronic obstructive pulmonary disease. *J Cardiopulm Rehabil* 22 (6): 426-430.

46. Engstrom, C.P., et al. 1999. Long-term effects of a pulmonary rehabilitation programme in outpatients with chronic obstructive pulmonary disease: A randomized controlled study. *Scand J Rehabil Med* 31 (4): 207-213.

47. Faglio, K., Bianchi, L., Ambrosino, N. 2001. Is it really useful to repeat outpatient pulmonary rehabilitation programs in patients with chronic airway obstruction? A 2-year controlled study. *Chest* 119 (6): 1696-1704.

48. Bauldoff, G.S., Hoffman, L.A., Zullo., T.G., and Sciurba, F.C. 2002. Exercise maintenance following pulmonary rehabilitation: Effect of distractive stimuli. *Chest* 122 (3): 948-954.

49. Berry, M.J., et al. 2003. A randomized controlled trial comparing long-term and short-term exercise in patients with chronic obstructive pulmonary disease. *J Cardiopulm Rehab* 23 (1): 60-68.

50. Wijkstra, P.J., and Strijbos, J.H. 1998. Home-based rehabilitation for patients with chronic obstructive pulmonary disease. *Monaldi Arch Chest Dis* 53 (4): 450-453.

51. Brooks, D., Krip, B., Mangovski-Alzamora, S., and Goldstein, R.S. 2002. The effect of postrehabilitation programmes among individuals with chronic obstructive pulmonary disease. *Eur Respir J* 20: 20-29.

52. Marlatt, G.A., and Gordon, J.R., eds. 1985. *Relapse prevention: Maintenance strategies in the treatment of addictive behaviors*. New York: Guilford.

53. Ries., A.L., Kaplan, R.M., Myers, R., and Prewitt, L.M. 2003. Maintenance after pulmonary rehabilitation in chronic lung disease. *Am J Respir Crit Care Med* 167: 880-888.

Chapter 6

1. Anon. 1999. Pulmonary rehabilitation—1999. The official statement of the American Thoracic Society. *Am J Respir Crit Care Med* 159: 1666-1682.

2. Jones, P.W. 1997. Quality of life measurements: The value of standardization. *Eur Respir Rev* 7: 46-49.

3. Carr, A.J., Gibson, B., and Robinson, P.G. 2001. Measuring quality of life: Is quality of life determined by expectations or experience? *BMJ* 322: 1240-1243.

4. Guyatt, G.H., Berman, L.B., Townsend, M., Pugsley, S.O., and Chambers, L.W. 1987. A measure of quality of life for clinical trials in chronic lung disease. *Thorax* 42: 773-778.

5. Williams, J.E., Singh, S.J., Sewell, L., and Morgan, M.D. 2003. Health status measurement: Sensitivity of the self-reported Chronic Respiratory Questionnaire (CRQ-SR) in pulmonary rehabilitation. *Thorax* 58 (6): 515-518.

6. Ware, J.E. 1993. *Health survey manual and interpretation guide*. Boston: The Health Institute, New England Medical Center.

7. Borg, G.A.V. 1982. Psychophysical bases of perceived exertion. *Med Sci Sports Exerc* 14: 377-381.

8. Reardon, J., Awad, E., Normandin, E., Vale, F., Clark, B., and ZuWallack, R.L. 1994. The effect of comprehensive outpatient pulmonary rehabilitation on dyspnea. *Chest* 105: 1046-1052.

9. Mahler, D., Guyatt, G., and Jones, P. 1998 Clinical measurement of dyspnea. In *Pulmonary rehabilitation: Lung biology in health and disease: Dyspnea*, vol. 111. Edited by D. Mahler, 149-198. New York: Marcel Decker.

10. Mahler, D.A., Weinberg, D.H., Wells, C.K., and Feinstein, A. 1984. The measurement of dyspnea: Contents, interobserver agreement, and physiologic correlations of two new clinical indexes. *Chest* 85: 751-758.

11. Eakin, E.G., Resnikoff, P.M., Prewitt, L.M., Ries, A.L., and Kaplan, R.M. 1998. Validation of a new dyspnea measure: The UCSD shortness of breath questionnaire. *Chest* 113: 619-624.

12. Fletcher, C.M. 1952. The clinical diagnosis of pulmonary emphysema: An experimental study. *Proc R Soc Med* 45: 577-584.

13. Fletcher, C.M., Elmes, P.C., and Wood, C.H. 1959. The significance of respiratory symptoms and the diagnosis of chronic bronchitis in a working population. *Br Med J* 2: 257-266.

14. Weaver, T.E., and Narsavage, G.L. 1992. Physiological and psychological variables related to functional status in chronic obstructive pulmonary disease. *Nurs Res* 41: 286-291.

15. Lareau, S., Carrieri-Kohlman, V., Janson-Bjerklie, S., and Roos, P.J. 1994. Development and testing of the pulmonary functional status and dyspnea questionnaire (PFSDQ). *Heart & Lung* 23: 242-250.

16. Lareau, S.C., Meek, P.M., and Roos, P.J. 1998. Development and testing of the modified version of the pulmonary functional status and dyspnea questionnaire (PFSDQ-M). *Heart & Lung* 27: 159-168.

17. Singh, S.J., Morgan, M.D., Scott, S., Walters, D., and Hardman, A.E. 1992. Development of a shuttle walking test of disability in patients with chronic airways obstruction. *Thorax* 47 (12): 1019-1024.

18. Revill, S.M., Morgan, M.D., Singh, S.J., Williams, J., and Hardman, A.E. 1999. The endurance shuttle walk: A new field test for the assessment of endurance capacity in chronic obstructive pulmonary disease. *Thorax* 54 (3): 213-222.

Chapter 7

1. American Thoracic Society and European Respiratory Society. 1999. Statement: Skeletal muscle dysfunction in COPD. *Am J Respir Crit Care Med* 159: S1-S40.

2. Decramer, M., Gosselink, R., Troosters, T., Verschuieren, M., and Evers, G. 1997. Muscle weakness is related to utilization of health care resources in COPD patients. *Eur Respir J* 10: 417-423.

3. Gray-Donald, K., Gibbons, L., Shapiro, S.H., Macklem, P.T., and Martin, J.G. 1996. Nutritional status and mortality in chronic obstructive pulmonary disease. *Am J Respir Crit Care Med* 153: 961-966.

4. Foster, S., and Thomas, H.M., III. 1990. Pulmonary rehabilitation in lung disease other than chronic obstructive pulmonary disease. *Am Rev Respir Dis* 141: 601-604.

5. Bach, J.R. 1993. Pulmonary rehabilitation. In *Rehabilitation medicine principles and pulmonary practice,* J.D. Delisa, ed. 952-972. Philadelphia: Lippincott.

6. Bach, J.R. 1993. Mechanical exsufflation, noninvasive ventilation, and new strategies for pulmonary rehabilitation and sleep disordered breathing. *NY Acad Med* 68: 321-340.

7. Bach, J.R. 1993. Pulmonary rehabilitation in neuromuscular disorders. *Neurology* 14: 515-529.

8. Novitch, R.S., and Thomas, H.M., III. 1995. Pulmonary rehabilitation in patients with interstitial lung disease. *Am Rev Respir Dis* 152: A684.

9. Cowley, R.S., et al. 1994. The role of rehabilitation in the intensive care unit. *J Head Trauma Rehabil* 9 (1): 32-42.

10. Satta, A. 2000. Exercise training in asthma. *J Sports Med Phys Fitness* 40 (4): 277-283.

11. Clark, C.J. 1993. The role of physical training in asthma. In *Principles and practice of pulmonary rehabilitation,* R. Casaburi and T. Petty, eds. 424-438. Philadelphia: Saunders.

12. Kitsantas, A., and Zimmerman, B.J. 2000. Self-efficacy, activity participation, and physical fitness of asthmatic and nonasthmatic adolescent girls. *J Asthma* 37 (2): 163-174.

13. Apter, A.J., Reisine, S.T., Affleck, G., Barrows, E., and ZuWallack, R. 1999. The influence of demographic and socioeconomic factors on health related quality of life in asthma. *Journal of Allergy & Clinical Immunol* 107: 27-78.

14. Dyer, C.A.E., Hill, S.L., Stockley, R.A., and Sinclair, A.J. 1999. Quality of life in elderly subjects with a diagnostic label of asthma from general practice registers. *Eur Respir J* 14: 39-45.

15. Emter, M., Herala, M., and Stalenheim, G. 1996. High-intensity physical training in adults with asthma: A 10-week rehabilitation program. *Chest* 109: 323-330.

16. Folgering, H., and Herwaarden, C.V. 1993. Pulmonary rehabilitation in asthma and COPD: Physiologic basics. *Respir Med* 87 (Suppl. B): 41-44.

17. National Institutes of Health. 1997. *Asthma guidelines.*

18. Make, B. 1994. Collaborative self-management strategies for patients with respiratory disease. *Respir Care* 39: 566-579.

19. Strunk, R.C., et al. 1991. Rehabilitation of a patient with asthma in the outpatient setting. *J Allergy Clin Immunol* 87: 601-611.

20. Cochrane, L.M., and Clark, C.J. 1990. Benefits and problems of a physical training program for asthmatic patients. *Thorax* 45: 345-351.

21. Cambach, W., Wagenaar, R.C., Koelman, T.W., Ton van Keimpema, A.R.J., and Kemper, H.C.G. 1999. The long-term effects of pulmonary rehabilitation in patients with asthma and chronic obstructive pulmonary disease: A research synthesis. *Arch Phys Med Rehabil* 80: 103-111.

22. Emter, M., Finne, M., and Stalenheim, G. 1998. High-intensity physical training in adults with asthma: A comparison between training on land and in water. *Scand J Rehabil Med* 30: 201-209.

23. Matsumoto, I., Araki, H., Tsuda, K., Odajima, H., Nishima, S., Higaki, Y., Tanaka, H., Tanaka, M., and Shindo, M. 1999. Effects of swimming training on aerobic capacity and exercise-induced bronchoconstriction in children with bronchial asthma. *Thorax* 54: 196-201.

24. Hallstrand, T.S., Bates, P.W., and Schoene, R.B. 2000. Aerobic conditioning in mild asthma decreases the hyperpnea of exercise and improves exercise and ventilatory capacity. *Chest* 118 (5): 1460-1469.

25. Neder, J.A., Nery, L.E., Silva, A.C., Cabral, A.L.B., and Fernandes, A.L.G. 1999. Short-term effects of aerobic training in the clinical management of moderate to severe asthma in children. *Thorax* 54: 202-206.

26. Emter, M., Finne, M., and Stalenheim, G. 1998. A 3-

year follow-up of asthmatic patients participating in a 10-week rehabilitation program with emphasis on physical training. *Arch Phys Med Rehabil* 79: 539-544.

27. Holloway, E., and Ram, F.S. 2004. Breathing exercises for asthma. *Cochrane Review.* In The Cochrane Library, issue 2. Chichester, U.K.: John Wiley & Sons, LTD.

28. Cox, N.J.M., Hendricks, J.C., Binkhorst, R.A., and van Herwaarden, C.L.A. 1993. A pulmonary rehabilitation program for patients with asthma and mild chronic obstructive pulmonary disease. *Lung* 171: 235-244.

29. FitzSimmons, S. 1993. The changing epidemiology of cystic fibrosis. *J Paediatr* 122: 1-9.

30. Scanlin, T. 1988. Cystic fibrosis. In *Pulmonary diseases and disorders*, 2nd ed. Edited by A. Fishman, 1273-1294. New York: McGraw-Hill.

31. McKone, E.F., Barry, S.C., Fitzgerald, M.X., and Gallagher, C.G. 2002. The role of supplemental oxygen during submaximal exercise in patients with cystic fibrosis. *Eur Respir J* 20: 134-142.

32. Nixon, P.A. 1996. Role of exercise in the evaluation and management of pulmonary disease in children and youth. *Med Sci Sports Exerc* 28 (4): 414-420.

33. Orenstein, D.M., and Noyes, B.E. 1993. Cystic fibrosis. In *Principles and practice of pulmonary rehabilitation*, R. Casaburi and T. Petty, eds. 439-458. Philadelphia: Saunders.

34. Murphy, S. 1987. Cystic fibrosis in adults: Diagnosis and management. *Clin Chest Med* 8: 695-710.

35. Moorcroft, A.J., Dodd, M.E., and Webb, A.K. 1998. Exercise limitations and training for patients with cystic fibrosis. *Disabil and Rehabil* 20 (6,7): 247-253.

36. Boas, S.R. 1997. Exercise recommendations for individuals with cystic fibrosis. *Sports Med* July 24 (1): 17-37.

37. Moorcroft, A.J., Dodd, M.E., and Webb, A.K. 1994. Exercise testing and prognosis in adult cystic fibrosis (Abstract). *Thorax* 49: 1075p-1076p.

38. Nixon, P.A., Orenstein, D.M., Kelsey, S.F., and Doershuk, C.F. 1992. The prognostic value of exercise testing in patients with cystic fibrosis. *New Engl J Med* 327: 1785-1788.

39. Prasad, S.A., Tannenbaum, E.L., and Mikelsons, C. 2000. Physiotherapy in cystic fibrosis. *J R Soc Med* 93 (Suppl. 38): 27-36.

40. Bradley, J., and Moran, F. 2004. Physical training for cystic fibrosis. *Cochrane Review.* In *The Cochrane Library,* issue 2. Chichester, U.K.: John Wiley & Sons, LTD.

41. Blau, H., Mussaffi-Georgy, H., Fink, G., Kaye, C., Szeinberg, A., Spitzer, S.A., and Yahav, J. 2002. Effects of an intensive 4-week summer camp on cystic fibrosis: Pulmonary function, exercise tolerance and nutrition. *Chest* 121: 1117-1122.

42. Gulmans, V.A.M., de Meer, K., Brackel, H.J.L., Faber, J.A.J., Berger, R., and Helders, P.J.M. 1999. Outpatient exercise training in children with cystic fibrosis: Physiological effects, perceived competence and acceptability. *Pediatr Pulmonol* 28: 39-46.

43. Strauss, G.D., Osher, A., Wang, C.I., Goodrich, E., Gold, F., Colman, W., Stabile, M., Dobrenchuk, A., and Keens, T.G. 1987. Variable weight training in cystic fibrosis. *Chest* 92 (2): 273-276.

44. Schneiderman-Walker, J., Pollock, S.L., Corey, M., Wilkes, D.D., Canny, G.J., Pedder, L., and Reisman, J.J. 2000. A randomized controlled trial of a 3-year home exercise program in cystic fibrosis. *J Pediatr* 136: 304-310.

45. Frangolias, D.D., Holloway, C.L., Vedal, S., and Wilcox, P.G. 2003. Role of exercise and lung function in predicting work status in cystic fibrosis. *Am J Respir Crit Care Med* 167: 150-157.

46. Cooper, D.M. 1998. Exercise and cystic fibrosis: The search for a therapeutic optimum. *Pediatr Pulm* 25: 43-44.

47. Asher, M.I., Pardy, R.L., Coates, A.L., Thomas, E., and Macklem, P.T. 1982. The effect of inspiratory muscle training in patients with cystic fibrosis. *Am Rev Respir Dis* 126: 855-859.

48. de Jong, W., van Aalderen, W.M., Kraan, J., Koeter, G.H., and van der Schans, C.P. 2001. Inspiratory muscle training in patients with cystic fibrosis. *Respir Med* 95 (1): 31-36.

49. Sawyer, E.H., and Clanton, T.L. 1993. Improved pulmonary function and exercise tolerance with inspiratory muscle conditioning in children with cystic fibrosis. *Chest* 104: 1490-1497.

50. Shepherd, R.W., and Cleghorn, G.J. 1989. Nutritional management. In *Cystic fibrosis: Nutritional and intestinal disorders,* R.W. Sheperd, ed. 53-65. Boca Raton, FL: CRC Press.

51. Luder, E. 1991. Nutritional care of patients with cystic fibrosis. *Top Clin Nutr* 6: 39-50.

52. Daniels, L.A., and Davidson, G.P. 1989. Current issues in the nutritional management of children with cystic fibrosis. *Aust Paediatr J* 25: 261-266.

53. Heijerman, H.G.M. 1993. Chronic obstructive lung disease and respiratory muscle function: The role of nutrition and exercise training in cystic fibrosis. *Respir Med* 87 (Suppl. B): 49-51.

54. American Thoracic Society and European Respiratory Society. 2000. Joint statement. Idiopathic pulmonary fibrosis: Diagnosis and treatment. International consensus statement. *Am J Respir Crit Care Med* 161: 646-664.

55. Fulmer, J.D. 1990. Interstitial lung diseases. In *Internal medicine,* 2nd ed. Edited by J.H. Stein, 675-683. Norwalk, CT: Appleton & Lange.

56. King, T.E., Jr., Cherniac, R.M., and Schwarz, M.I. 1994. Idiopathic pulmonary fibrosis and other interstitial lung disease of unknown etiology. In *Textbook of respiratory medicine*, vol. 2. Edited by J.F. Murray and J.A. Nadel, 287-303. Philadelphia: Saunders.

57. Chang, J.A., Curtis, J.R., Patrick, D.L., and Raghu, G. 1999. Assessment of health-related quality of life in patients with interstitial lung disease. *Chest* 116: 1175-1182.

58. DeVries, J., Kessels, B.L., and Drent, M. 2001. Quality of life of idiopathic pulmonary fibrosis. *Eur Respir J* 17 (5): 954-961.

59. Martinez, T.Y., Pereira, C.A., dos Santos, M.L., Ciconelli, R.M., Guimaraes, S.M., and Martinez, J.A. 2000. Evaluation of the short-form 36-item questionnaire to measure health-related quality of life in patients with idiopathic pulmonary fibrosis. *Chest* 117 (6): 1627-1632.

60. Harris-Eze, A.O., Sridhar, G., Clemens, R.E., Zintel, T.A., Gallagher, C.G., and Marciniuk, D.D. 1996. Role of hypoxemia and pulmonary mechanics in exercise limitation in interstitial lung disease. *Am J Respir Crit Care Med* 154: 994-1001.

61. Markovitz, G.H., and Cooper, C.B. 1998. Exercise and interstitial lung disease. *Curr Opin Pulm Med* 4: 272-280.

62. Marciniuk, D.D, Sridhar, G., Clemens, R.E., Zintel, T.A., and Gallagher, C.G. 1994. Lung volumes and expiratory flow limitation during exercise in interstitial lung disease. *J Appl Physiol* 77 (2): 963-973.

63. Hansen, J.E., and Wasserman, K. 1996. Pathophysiology of activity limitation in patients with interstitial lung disease. *Chest* 109: 1566-1576.

64. O'Donnell, D.E., Chau, L.K.L., and Webb, K.A. 1998. Qualitative aspects of exertional dyspnea in patients with interstitial lung disease. *J Appl Physiol* 84 (6): 2000-2009.

65. Hsia, C.C.W. 1999. Cardiopulmonary limitations to exercise in restrictive lung disease. *Med Sci Sports Exerc* 31 (1 Suppl.): S28-S32.

66. Novitch, R.S., and Thomas, H.M., III. 1996. Pulmonary rehabilitation in chronic pulmonary interstitial disease. In *Pulmonary rehabilitation: Lung biology in health and disease*, vol. 91. Edited by A.P. Fishman, 683-700. New York: Marcel Dekker.

67. Siegler, E.L., Stineman, M.G., and Maislin, G. 1994. Development of complications during rehabilitation. *Arch Intern Med* 145: 2185-2190.

68. Nonn, R.A., and Garrity, E.R. 1998. Lung transplantation for fibrotic lung diseases. *Am J Med Sci* 315 (3): 146-154.

69. Foster, S., and Thomas, H.M., III. 1990. Pulmonary rehabilitation in lung disease other than chronic obstructive pulmonary disease. *Am Rev Respir Dis* 141: 601-604.

70. Marciniuk, D.D., and Gallagher, C.G. 1994. Clinical exercise testing in interstitial lung disease. *Clin Chest Med* 15 (2): 287-303.

71. Harris-Eze, A.O., Sridhar, G., Clemens, R.E., Gallagher, C.G., and Marciniuk, D.D. 1994. Oxygen improves maximal exercise performance in interstitial lung disease. *Am J Respir Crit Care Med* 150: 1616-1622.

72. Jakicic, J.M., Clark, K., Coleman, E., Donnelly, J.E., Foreyt, J., Melanson, E., Volek, J., and Volpe, S.L. 2001. Appropriate intervention strategies for weight loss and prevention of weight regain for adults. *Med Sci Sports Exerc* 33 (12): 2145-2156.

73. World Health Organization. 1997. Obesity: Preventing and managing the global epidemic. Report of a WHO consultation on obesity. Geneva, June 3-5.

74. Stevens, J., Cai, J., Pamuk, E.R., Williamson, D.F., Thun, M.J., and Wood, J.L. 1998. The effect of age on the association between body mass index and mortality. *New Engl J Med* 338: 1-7.

75. Pi-Sunyer, F.X. 1993. Medical hazards of obesity. *Ann Intern Med* 119: 655-60.

76. Miller, W.C. 2001. Effective diet and exercise treatments for overweight and recommendations for intervention. *Sports Med* 31 (10): 717-724.

77. Luce, J.M. 1980. Respiratory complications of obesity. *Chest* 78 (4): 626-631.

78. Koenig, S.M. 2001. Pulmonary complications of obesity. *Am J Med Sci* 321 (4): 249-279.

79. Mohsenin, V., and Gee, J.B.L. 1993. Effect of obesity on the respiratory system and pathophysiology of sleep apnea. *Curr Pulmonol* 14: 179-197.

80. Strollo, P.J., and Rogers, R.M. 1996. Obstructive sleep apnea. *New Engl J Med* 334 (2): 99-104.

81. Fontaine, K.R., and Barofsky, I. 2001. Obesity and health-related quality of life. *Obesity Reviews* 2 (3): 173-182.

82. Larsson, U.E., and Mattsson, E. 2001. Perceived disability and observed functional limitations in obese women. *Int J Obes Rel Metab Dis* 259 (11): 1705-1712.

83. Lean, M.E., Han, J.S., and Seidelo, J.C. 1999. Impairment of health and quality of life using new vs. federal guidelines for the identification of obesity. *Arch Intern Med* 159 (8): 837-843.

84. Wasserman, K., Hansen, J.E., Sue, D.Y., Casaburi, R., and Whipp, B.J., eds. 1999. *Principles of exercise testing and interpretation*, 3rd ed., 272-277. Philadelphia: Lippincott, Williams, & Wilkins.

85. Alpert, M.A., Singh, A., Terry, B.E., Kelly, D.L., Sharaf El-Deane, M.S., Mukerji, V., Villarereal, D., and Artis, A.K. 1989. Effect of exercise and cavity size on right ventricular function in morbid obesity. *Am J Cardiol* 64: 1361-1365.

86. Pratley, R.E., Hagberg, J.M., Dengel, D.R., Rogus, E.M., Muller, D.C., and Goldberg, A.P. 2000. Aerobic

exercise training-induced reductions in abdominal fat and glucose-stimulated insulin responses in middle-aged and older men. *J Am Ger Soc* 48 (9): 1055-1061.

87. Hakala, K., Mustajdki, P., Aittomaki, J., and Sovijarvi, A. 1996. Improved gas exchange during exercise after weight loss in morbid obesity. *Clin Physiol* 16: 229-238.

88. Weiner, P., Waizman, J., Weiner, M., Rabner, M., Magadle, R., and Zamir, D. 1998. Influence of excessive weight loss after gastroplasty for morbid obesity on respiratory muscle performance. *Thorax* 53: 39-42.

89. Hakala, K., Mustajoiki, P., Aittomaki, J., and Sovijarvi, A. 2000. Improved gas exchange during exercise after weight loss in morbid obesity. *Clin Physiol* 16: 229-238.

90. Rubenstein, I., Colapinto, N., Rosstein, L.E., Brown, I.G., and Hoffstein, V. 1988. Improvement in upper airway function after weight loss in patients with observeable sleep apnea. *Am Rev Respir Dis* 178: 1192-1195.

91. Sugerman, H.J., Fairman, R.P., Lindeman, A.K., Mathers, J.A.L., and Greenfield, L.J. 1981. Gastroplasty for respiratory insufficiency of obesity. *Ann Surg* 193 (6): 677-683.

92. Kanoupakis, E., Michaloudis, D., Fraidakis, O., Patrhenakis, F., Vardas, P., and Melissas, J. 2001. Left ventricular function and cardiopulmonary performance following surgical treatment of morbid obesity. *Obesity Surg* 11 (5): 552-558.

93. Collazo-Clavell, M.A. 1999. Safe and effective management of the obese patient. *Mayo Clin Proc* 74: 1255-1260.

94. Pate, R.R., Pratt, M., Blair, S.N., Haskell, W.L., Macera, C., Bouchard, C., et al. 1995. Physical activity and public health. A recommendation for the Centers for Disease Control and Prevention and the American College of Sports Medicine. *JAMA* 273: 402-407.

95. Ross, R., Dagnone, D., Jones, P.J.H., Smith, H., Paddags, A., Hudson, R., and Janssen, I. 2000. Reduction in obesity and related comorbid conditions after diet-induced weight loss or exercise-induced weight loss in men: A randomized controlled trial. *Ann Intern Med* 133: 92-103.

96. Knipper, J., Nielsen, N., Lane-Gipson, N., Maxwell, G., Muller, D., Wilson, J., and Geist, L. 2000. Outcomes of pulmonary rehabilitation in obstructive sleep apnea (Abstract). *Am J Respir Crit Care Med*: A496.

97. Whittaker, L.A., Brodeur, L.E., and Rochester, C.L. 2000. Functional outcome of inpatient pulmonary rehabilitation for patients with morbid obesity (Abstract). *Am J Respir Crit Care Med* March 2000: A495.

98. Guernelli, J., Wainapel, S.F., Pack, S., and Miranda-Lama, E. 1999. Morbidly-obese patients with pulmonary disease: A retrospective study of four cases. *Am J Phys Med Rehabil* 78: 60-65.

99. Ravens-Sieberer, U., Redegeld, Z.M., and Bullinger, M. 2001. Quality of life after inpatient rehabilitation in children with obesity. *Int J Obes Rel Metab Dis* 25 (Suppl. 1): S63-S65.

100. Matthay, R.A., and Matthay, M.A. 1990. Pulmonary thromboembolism and other pulmonary vascular diseases. In *Chest medicine: Essentials of pulmonary and critical care medicine*, 2nd ed. Edited by R.B. George, R.W. Light, M.A. Matthay, and R.A. Matthay, 249-276. Baltimore: Williams & Wilkins.

101. Rich, S., Dantzker, D.R., Ayres, S.M., et al. 1987. Primary pulmonary hypertension: A national prospective study. *Ann Intern Med* 107: 216.

102. Palevsky, H.I. 1997. Therapeutic options for severe pulmonary hypertension. *Clin Chest Med* 18 (3): 595-609.

103. Wasserman, K., et al. 1999. Pathophysiology of disorders limiting exercise. In *Principles of exercise testing and interpretation*, 3rd ed. Edited by K. Wasserman, J.E. Hansen, D.Y. Sue, R. Casaburi, and B.J. Whipp, 272-277. Philadelphia: Lippincott Williams & Wilkins.

104. American College of Chest Physicians and National Heart, Lung and Blood Institute National Conference on oxygen therapy. 1984. *Chest* 86: 234.

105. Rubin, L.J. 2003. Prognosis and treatment of primary pulmonary hypertension. www.uptodate.com. Accessed April 25, 2003.

106. Rogers, T.K., and Howard, P. 1992. Pulmonary hemodynamics and physical training in patients with chronic obstructive pulmonary disease. *Chest* 101: 289S.

107. Hill, N.S., and Lynch J.P., 2002. Pulmonary complications of neuromuscular diseases. *Semin Respir Crit Care Med* 23 (3): 189-314.

108. Fanburg, B.L., and Sicilian, L., eds. 1994. Respiratory dysfunction in neuromuscular disease. *Clin Chest Med* 15 (4): 607-810.

109. Bach, J.R., and Alba, A.S. 1991. Pulmonary dysfunction and sleep disordered breathing as post-polio sequelae: Evaluation and management. *Orthopedics* 14: 1329-1337.

110. Brooke, M.H., et al. 1989. Duchenne muscular dystrophy: Patterns of clinical progression and effects of supportive therapy. *Neurology* 39: 475-481.

111. Bach, J.R., Campagnolo, D.I., and Hoeman, S. 1991. Life satisfaction of individuals with Duchenne muscular dystrophy using long-term mechanical ventilatory support. *Am J Phys Med Rehabil* 70: 129-135.

112. Bach, J.R. 1992. Pulmonary rehabilitation considerations for Duchenne muscular dystrophy: The prolongation of life by respiratory muscle aids. *Crit Rev Phys Rehabil Med* 3: 239-269.

113. Silver, J.K., and Aiello, D.D. 2002. What internists need to know about post-polio syndrome. *Cleve Clin J Med* 69 (9): 704-712.

114. Bach, J.R. 1996. Conventional approaches to managing neuromuscular ventilatory failure. In *Pulmonary rehabilitation: The obstructive and paralytic conditions,* J.R. Bach, ed. 285-303.

115. Ansved, T. 2001. Muscle training in muscular dystrophies. *Acta Physiol Scand* 171: 359-366.

116. de Goede, C.J.T., Keus, S.H.J., Kwakkel, G., and Wagenaar, R.C. 2001. The effects of physical therapy in Parkinson's disease: A research synthesis. *Arch Phys Med Rehabil* 82: 509-515.

117. Baatile, J., Langbein, W.E., Weaver, F., Maloney, C., and Jost, M.B. 2000. Effect of exercise on perceived quality of life of individuals with Parkinson's disease. *J Rehabil Res Devel* 37 (5): 529-534.

118. O'Hara, L., and Ide, L. 2000. Physical rehabilitation has a positive effect on disability in multiple sclerosis patients. *Neurology* 54: 1396-1397.

119. Drory, V.E., Goltsman, E., Reznik, J.G., Mosek, A., and Korczyn, A.D. 2001. The value of muscle exercise in patients with amyotrophic lateral sclerosis. *J Neurol Sci* 191: 133-137.

120. Kilmer, D.D., Aitkens, S.G., Wright, N.C., and McCrory, M.A. 2001. Response to high-intensity eccentric muscle contractions in persons with myopathic disease. *Muscle and Nerve* 24: 1181-1187.

121. Philips, B.A., and Mastaglia, F.L. 2000. Exercise therapy in patients with myopathy. *Curr Opin Neurol* 13: 547-552.

122. Agre, J.C., and Sliwa, J.A. 2000. Neuromuscular rehabilitation and electrodiagnosis. 4. Specialized neuropathy. *Arch Phys Med Rehabil* 81: S27-S31.

123. Baydur, A., Layne, E., Aral, H., Krishnareddy, N., Topacio, R., Frederick, G., and Bodden, W. 2000. Long-term non-invasive ventilation in the community for patients with musculoskeletal disorders: 46-year experience and review. *Thorax* 55: 4-11.

124. American Association for Respiratory Care. 1991. Postural drainage therapy. *Respir Care* 36 (12): 1418.

125. Kigin, C.M. 1990. Breathing exercises for the medical patient: The art and the science. *Phys Ther* 70: 700-706.

126. Koessler, W., Wanke, T., Winkler, G., Nader, A., Toifl, K., Kurz, H., and Zwick, H. 2001. Two years' experience with inspiratory muscle training in patients with neuromuscular disorders. *Chest* 120: 765-769.

127. Unterburn, J.N., and Hill, N.S. 1994. Options for mechanical ventilation on neuromuscular diseases. *Clin Chest Med* 15: 765-781.

128. Schneerson, J.M. 1998. Rehabilitation in neuromuscular disorders and thoracic wall deformities. *Monaldi Arch Chest Dis* 53 (4): 415-418.

129. ATS guidelines: Lung volume reduction surgery. 2003. www.uptodate.com. Accessed April 28, 2003.

130. Flaherty, K.R., and Martinez, F.J. 2000. Lung volume reduction surgery for emphysema. *Clin Chest Med* 21: 819-848.

131. Cordova, F.C., and Criner, G.J. 2001. Surgery for chronic obstructive pulmonary disease: The place for lung volume reduction and transplantation. *Curr Opin Pulm Med* 7 (2): 93-104.

132. National Emphysema Treatment Trial Research Group. 2000. Rationale and design of the National Emphysema Treatment Trial: A prospective randomized trial of lung volume reduction surgery. *J Cardiopulm Rehabil* 20 (1): 24-36.

133. Geddes, D., Davies, M., Koyama, H., Hansell, D., Pastorino, U., Pepper, J., Agent, P., Cullinan, P., MacNeill, S.J., and Goldstraw, P. 2000. Effect of lung volume reduction surgery in patients with severe emphysema. *N Engl J Med* 343: 239-245.

134. Gelb, A.F., McKenna, R.J., Jr., Brenner, M., Epstein, J.D., and Zamel, N. 2001. Lung function 5 years after lung volume reduction surgery. *Am J Respir Crit Care Med* 163: 1562-1566.

135. Wilkens, H., Demertzis, S., Konig, J., Leitnaker, C.K., Schafers, H.J., and Sybrecht, G.W. 2000. Lung reduction surgery versus conservative treatment in severe emphysema. *Eur Respir J* 16: 1043-1049.

136. Cooper, J.D., Patterson, G.A., Sundaresan, R.S., et al. 1996. Results of 150 consecutive bilateral lung volume reduction procedures in patients with severe emphysema. *J Thorac Cardiovasc Surg* 111: 310-322.

137. Gelb, A.F., McKenna, R.J., Jr., Brenner, M., Schein, M.J., Zamel, N., and Fischel, R. 1999. Lung function 4 years after lung volume reduction surgery for emphysema. *Chest* 116: 1608-1615.

138. Sciurba, F.C., et al. 1996. Improvement in pulmonary function and elastic recoil after lung reduction surgery. *N Engl J Med* 334: 1095-1099.

139. Teschler, H., Stomatis, G., and Forhat, A.A.E. 1996. Effect of lung volume reduction surgery on respiratory muscle function in pulmonary emphysema. *Eur Respir J* 9: 1779-1784.

140. Leyenson, V., Furukawa, S., Kuzma, A.M., Cordova, F., Travaline, J., and Criner, G.J. 2000. Correlation of changes in quality of life after lung volume reduction surgery with changes in lung function, exercise and gas exchange. *Chest* 118: 728-735.

141. Mineo, T.C., Pompeo, E., Rogliani, P., Dauri, M., Turani, F., Bollero, P., and Magliocchetti, N. 2002. Effect of lung volume reduction surgery for severe emphysema on right ventricular function. *Am J Respir Crit Care Med* 165: 489-494.

142. Celli, B.R., Montes de Oca, M., Mendez, R., and Stetz, J. 1997. Lung reduction surgery decreases central drive and ventilatory response to CO_2. *Chest* 112: 902.

143. National Emphysema Treatment Trial Research Group. 2003. A randomized controlled trial comparing lung volume reduction surgery with medical therapy for severe emphysema. *N Engl J Med* 348 (21): 2059-2073.

144. National Emphysema Treatment Trial Research Group. 2001. Patients at high risk of death after lung-volume reduction surgery. *N Engl J Med* 345 (15): 1075-1083.

145. Criner, G.J., Cordova, F.C., Furukawa, S., Kuzma, A.M., Travaline, J.M., Leyenson, V., and O'Brien, G.M. 1999. Prospective randomized trial comparing bilateral lung volume reduction surgery to pulmonary rehabilitation in severe chronic obstructive pulmonary disease. *Am J Respir Crit Care Med* 160: 2018-2027.

146. American Thoracic Society and European Respiratory Society. 1998. International guidelines for selection of lung transplant candidates. *Am J Respir Crit Care Med* 158: 335-339.

147. Edelman, J.D., and Kotloff, R.M. 1997. Lung transplantation: A disease-specific approach. *Clin Chest Med* 18 (3): 627-644.

148. Steinman, T.I., Becker, B., Frost, A.E., Olthoff, K.M., Smart, F.W., Suki, W.N., and Wilkinson, A.H. 2001. Guidelines for the referral and management of patients eligible for solid organ transplantation. *Transplantation* 71 (9): 1189-1204.

149. Schulman, L.L. 2000. Lung transplantation for chronic obstructive pulmonary disease. *Clin Chest Med* 21: 849-865.

150. Cooper, J.D. 1990. Lung transplantation. *Heart and lung*. W.A. Baumgartner, B.A. Reitz, and S.C. Achuff, eds. 347-371. Philadelphia: Saunders.

151. Sheldon, J.B., et al. 1993. Pulmonary rehabilitation prior to lung transplantation. *Am Rev Respir Dis* 147: A597.

152. Niederman, M.S., et al. 1991. Benefits of a pulmonary rehabilitation program: Improvements are independent of lung function. *Chest* 99: 798-804.

153. Biggar, D., et al. 1993. Medium term results of pulmonary rehabilitation prior to lung transplantation. *Am Rev Respir Dis* 47 (4): A33.

154. Punzal, P.A., et al. 1991. Maximum intensity exercise training in patients with COPD. *Chest* 100: 618-623.

155. Biggar, D.G., Mallen, J., and Trulock, E.P. 1993. Pulmonary rehabilitation before and after transplantation. In *Principles and practice of pulmonary rehabilitation*, R. Casaburi and T. Petty, eds. 459-469. Philadelphia: Saunders.

156. Surgit, O., Ersoz, G., Gursel, Y., and Ersoz, S. 2001. Effects of exercise training on specific immune parameters in transplant recipients. *Transplant Proceedings* 33: 3298.

157. Orens, J.B., et al. 1995. Cardiopulmonary exercise testing following allogeneic lung transplantation for different underlying disease states. *Chest* 107: 144-149.

158. Otulana, B.A., Higenbottam, T.W., and Wallwork, J. 1992. Causes of exercise limitation after heart-lung transplantation. *J Heart Lung Transplant* 11: S244-S251.

159. Menard-Rothe, D., et al. 1997. Self-selected walking velocity for functional ambulation in patients with end-stage emphysema. *J Cardiopulm Rehabil* 17 (2): 85-91.

160. Jemal, A., Thomas, A., Murrary, T., and Thun, M. 2002. Cancer statistics. *Cancer J Clin* 52: 23-47.

161. Beckett, W.S. 1993. Epidemiology and etiology of lung cancer. *Clin Chest Med* 14 (1): 17-30.

162. Zang, E.A., and Wynder, E.L. 1996. Differences in lung cancer risk between men and women: Examination of the evidence. *J Natl Cancer Inst* 88: 183-192.

163. Shields, T.W. 1993. Surgical therapy for carcinoma of the lung. *Clin Chest Med* 14 (1): 121-147.

164. Flehinger, B.J., Kimmel, M., and Melamad, M.R. 1992. The effect of surgical treatment on survival in early lung cancer: Implications for screening. *Chest* 101: 1013.

165. Smetana, G.W. 2003. Evaluation of preoperative pulmonary risk. www.uptodate.com. Accessed April 28, 2003.

166. Hall, J.C., Tarala, R.A., Hall, J.L., et al. 1991. A multivariate analysis of the risk of pulmonary complications after laparotomy. *Chest* 99: 923.

167. Wilson, D.J. 1997. Pulmonary rehabilitation exercise program for high risk thoracic surgical patients. *Chest Surg Clin N Am* 7 (4): 697-706.

168. Lawrence, V.A., Hilsenbeck, S.G., Mulrow, C.D., et al. 1995. Incidence and hospital stay for cardiac and pulmonary complications after abdominal surgery. *J Gen Intern Med* 10: 671.

169. Pedersen, T. 1994. Complications and death following anesthesia. *Dan Med Bull* 41: 319.

170. Markos, J., Mullan, B.P., Hillman, D.R., et al. 1989. Preoperative assessment as a predictor or mortality and morbidity after lung resection. *Am Rev Respir Dis* 139: 902.

171. Kearney, D.J., Lee, T.H., Reilly, J.J., et al. 1994. Assessment of operative risk in patients undergoing lung resection. *Chest* 105: 753.

172. Pierce, R.J., Copland, J.M., Sharpe, K., et al. 1994. Preoperative risk evaluation for lung cancer resection: Predicted postoperative product as a predictor of surgical mortality. *Am J Respir Crit Care Med* 150: 947.

173. Smith, T.P., Kinasewitz, G.T., Tucker, W.Y., et al. 1984. Exercise capacity as a predictor of postthoracotomy morbidity. *Am Rev Respir Dis* 129: 730.

174. Walsh, G.L., Morice, R.C., Putnam, J.B., Jr., et al. 1994. Resection of lung cancer is justified in high risk patients selected by exercise oxygen consumption. *Ann Thorac Surg* 58: 704.

175. Bolliger, C.T., Jordan, P., Soler, M., et al. 1995. Exercise capacity as a predictor of postoperative complications in lung resection candidates. *Am J Respir Crit Care Med* 151: 1472.

176. deRose, J.J., Jr., Argenziano, M., El-Amir, N., et al. 1998. Lung reduction operation and resection of pulmonary nodules in patients with severe emphysema. *Ann Thorac Surg* 65: 314.

177. Brunelli, A., al Refai, M., Monteverde, M., et al. 2002. Stair climbing test predicts cardiopulmonary complications after lung resection. *Chest* 121: 1106-1110.

178. Warner, M.A., Offord, K.P., Warner, M.E., et al. 1989. Role of preoperative cessation of smoking and other factors in postoperative pulmonary complications: A blinded prospective study of coronary artery bypass patients. *Mayo Clin Proc* 64: 609.

179. Thomas, J.A., and McIntosh, J.M. 1994. Are incentive spirometry, intermittent positive pressure breathing, and deep breathing exercises effective in the prevention of postoperative pulmonary complications after upper abdominal surgery? A systematic overview and meta-analysis. *Phys Ther* 74: 3.

180. Schwieger, I., Gamulin, Z., Forster, A., et al. 1986. Absence of benefit of incentive spirometry in low risk patients undergoing elective cholecystectomy: A randomized study. *Chest* 89: 652.

181. Brusasco, V., and Fitting, J.W. 1996. Lung hyperinflation in airway obstruction. *Eur Respir J* 9: 2440.

182. Casaburi, R., Patessio, A., Ioli, F., Zanaboni, S., Donner, C.F., and Wasserman, K. 1991. Reductions in lactic acidosis and ventilation as a result of exercise training in patients with obstructive lung disease. *Am Rev Respir Dis* 143: 9-18.

183. Maltais, F., Leblanc, P., Jobin, J., et al. 1997. Intensity of training and physiologic adaptation in patients with chronic obstructive pulmonary disease. *Am J Respir Crit Care Med* 155: 555-561.

184. Bourjeily, G., and Rochester, C.L. 2000. Exercise training in chronic obstructive pulmonary disease. *Clin Chest Med* 21: 763-781.

185. van't Hul, A., Kwakkel, G., and Gosselink, R. 2002. The acute effects of noninvasive ventilatory support during exercise on exercise endurance and dyspnea in patients with chronic obstructive pulmonary disease: A systematic review. *J Cardiopulm Rehabil* 22: 290-297.

186. O'Donnell, D.E., Sanii, R., and Younes, M. 1998. Improvements in exercise endurance in patients with chronic airflow limitation using continuous positive airway pressure. *Am Rev Respir Dis* 138: 1510-1514.

187. Ambrosino, N. 2000. Exercise and noninvasive ventilatory support. *Monaldi Arch Chest Dis* 55 (3): 242-246.

188. Bianchi, L., Fogio, K., Vitacca, M., et al. 1998. Effects of proportional assist ventilation on exercise tolerance in COPD patients with chronic hypercapnia. *Eur Respir J* 11: 422-427.

189. Henke, K.G., Regnis, J.A., and Bye, P.T.P. 1993. Benefits of continuous positive airway pressure during exercise in cystic fibrosis and relationship to disease severity. *Am Rev Respir Dis* 148: 1272-1276.

190. Appendini, I. 2003. Proportion of assist ventilation: Back to the future? *Respiration* 70: 345-346.

191. Hernandez, P., Maltais, F., Gursahaney, A., LeBlanc, P., and Gottfried, S.B. 2001. Proportional assist ventilation may improve exercise performance in severe chronic obstructive pulmonary disease. *J Cardiopulm Rehabil* 21 (3): 135-142.

192. Polkey, M.I., Hawkins, P., Kyroussis, D., Ellum, S.G., Sherwood, R., and Moxham, J. 2000. Inspiratory pressure support prolongs exercise induced lactataemia in severe COPD. *Thorax* 55: 547-549.

193. Dolmage, T.E., and Goldstein, R.S. 1997. Proportional assist ventilation and exercise tolerance in subjects with COPD. *Chest* 111 (4): 948-954.

194. Keilty, S.E.J., Ponte, J., Fleming, T.A., et al. 1994. Effect of inspiratory pressure support on exercise tolerance and breathlessness in patients with severe stable chronic obstructive pulmonary disease. *Thorax* 49: 990-994.

195. Maltais, F., Reissmann, H., and Gottfried, S.B. 1995. Pressure support reduces inspiratory effort and dyspnea during exercise in chronic airflow obstruction. *Am J Respir Crit Care Med* 151: 1027-1033.

196. Hawkins, P., Johnson, L.C., Nikoletou, D., Hamnegard, C.H., Sherwood, R., and Polkey, M.I. 2002. Proportional assist ventilation as an aid to exercise training in severe chronic obstructive pulmonary disease. *Thorax* 57: 853-859.

197. Johnson, J.E., Gavin, D.J., and Adams-Dramiga, S. 2002. Effects of training with heliox and noninvasive positive pressure ventilation on exercise ability in patients with severe COPD. *Chest* 122: 464-472.

198. Bianchi, L., Foglio, K., Porta, R., Baiardi, P., Vitacca, M., and Ambrosino, N. 2002. Lack of additional effect of adjunct of assisted ventilation to pulmonary rehabilitation in mild COPD patients. *Respir Med* 96: 359-367.

199. Garrod, R., Mikelsons, C., Paul, E.A., and Wedzicha, J.A. 2000. Randomized controlled trial of domiciliary noninvasive positive pressure ventilation and physical training in severe chronic obstructive pulmonary disease. *Am J Respir Crit Care Med* 162: 1335-1341.

200. Ferris, G., Servera-Pieras, E., Vergara, P.B.S., Tzeng, A.C., Perez, M., Marin, J., and Bach, J.R. 2000. Kyphoscoliosis ventilatory insufficiency: Noninva-

sive management outcomes. *Am J Phys Med Rehabil* 79 (1): 24-29.

201. Tsuboi, T., Ohi, M., Chin, K., et al. 1997. Ventilatory support during exercise in patients with pulmonary tuberculosis sequelae. *Chest* 112: 1000-1007.

202. Make, B., et al. 1984. Rehabilitation of ventilator-dependent subjects with lung diseases: The concept and initial experience. *Chest* 86 (3): 358-365.

203. Jackson, N.C. 1991. Pulmonary rehabilitation for mechanically ventilated patient. *Crit Care Nurs Clin North Am* 3 (4): 365-591.

204. O'Donohue, W.J., et al. 1986. Long-term mechanical ventilation: Guidelines for management in the home and alternate sites. *Chest* 90: 1S-37S.

205. Make, B.J., and Gilmartin, M.E. 1991. Care of ventilator-assisted individuals in the home and alternate sites. *Respiratory care: A guide to clinical practice.* G.G. Burton, J.E. Hodgkin, and J.J. Ward, eds. 669-690. Philadelphia: Lippincott.

206. Pierson, D.J., and Kacmarek, R.M. 1993. Home ventilator care. In *Principles and practice of pulmonary rehabilitation*, R. Casaburi and T. Petty, eds. 274-288. Philadelphia: Saunders.

207. Rodriguez, O., Braun, L., and Rosenson, R.S. 2003. Components of cardiac rehabilitation and exercise prescription. www.uptodate.com. Accessed May 1, 2003.

208. Kao, A., and Loh, E. 2003. Cardiac rehabilitation in patients with heart failure. www.uptodate.com. Accessed May 1, 2003.

Appendix C

1. Wasserman, K., Hansen, J.E., Sue, D.Y., Casaburi, R., and Whipp, B.J. 1999. *Principles of exercise testing and interpretation,* 3rd edition. Philadelphia: Lippincott Williams & Wilkins.

2. Weisman, I.M., and Zeballos, R.J. 1994. An integrated approach to the interpretation of cardiopulmonary exercise testing. *Clin Chest Med* 15: 421-445.

3. Fletcher, G.F., Balady, G., Froelicher, V.F., Hartley, L.H., Haskell, W.L., and Pollock, M.L. 1995. Exercise standards: A statement for healthcare professionals from the American Heart Association: Writing group. *Circulation* 91: 580-615.

4. Pina, I.L., Balady, G.J., Hanson, P., Labovitz, A.J., Madonna, D.W., and Myers, J. 1995. Guidelines for clinical exercise testing laboratories: A statement for health care professionals from the Committee on Exercise and Cardiac Rehabilitation, American Heart Association. *Circulation* 91: 912-921.

5. Balke, B. 1963. A simple field test for the assessment of physical fitness. *CARI Report* 63: 18.

6. Cooper, K.H. 1968. A means of assessing maximal oxygen intake: Correlation between field and treadmill testing. *JAMA* 203: 201-204.

7. McGavin, C.R., Gupta, S.P., and McHardy, G.J.R. 1976. Twelve-minute walking test for assessing disability in chronic bronchitis. *BMJ* 1: 822-823.

8. Butland, R.J.A., Pang, J., Gross, E.R., Woodcock, A.A., and Geddes, D.M. 1982. Two-, six-, and 12-minute walking tests in respiratory disease. *BMJ* 284: 1607-1608.

9. Solway, S., Brooks, D., Lacasse, Y., and Thomas, S. 2001. A qualitative systematic overview of the measurement properties of functional walk tests used in the cardiorespiratory domain. *Chest* 119: 256-270.

10. Kadikar, A., Maurer, J., and Kesten, S. 1997. The six-minute walk test: A guide to assessment for lung transplantation. *J Heart Lung Transplant* 16: 313-319.

11. Holden, D.A., Rice, T.W., Stelmach, K., and Meeker, D.P. 1992. Exercise testing, 6-minute walk, and stair climb in the evaluation of patients at high risk for pulmonary resection. *Chest* 102: 1774-1779.

12. Sciurba, F.C., Rogers, R.M., Keenan, R.J., Slivka, W.A., Gorcsan, J., III, Ferson, P.F., Holbert, J.M., Brown, M.L., and Landreneau, R.J. 1996. Improvement in pulmonary function and elastic recoil after lung-reduction surgery for diffuse emphysema. *N Engl J Med* 334: 1095-1099.

13. Criner, G.J., Cordova, F.C., Furukawa, S., Kuzma, A.M., Travaline, J.M., Leyenson, V., and O'Brien, G.M. 1999. Prospective randomized trial comparing bilateral lung volume reduction surgery to pulmonary rehabilitation in severe COPD. *Am J Respir Crit Care Med* 160: 2018-2027.

14. Sinclair, D.J.M., and Ingram, C.G. 1980. Controlled trial of supervised exercise training in chronic bronchitis. *BMJ* 280: 519-521.

15. Roomi, J., Johnson, M.M., Waters, K., Yohannes, A., Helm, A., and Connolly, M.J. 1996. Respiratory rehabilitation, exercise capacity, and quality of life in chronic airways disease in old age. *Age Ageing* 25: 12-16.

16. Paggiaro, P.L., Dahle, R., Bakran, I., Frith, L., Hollingworth, K., and Efthimiou, J. 1998. Multicentre randomized placebo-controlled trial of inhaled fluticasone propionate in patients with COPD. *Lancet* 351: 773-780.

17. Leggett, R.J., and Flenley, D.C. 1977. Portable oxygen and exercise tolerance in patients with chronic hypoxic cor pulmonale. *BMJ* 2: 84-86.

18. Spence, D.P.S., Hay, J.G., Carter, J., Pearson, M.G., and Calverley, P.M.A. 1993. Oxygen desaturation and breathlessness during corridor walking in COPD: Effect of oxitropium bromide. *Thorax* 48: 1145-1150.

19. DeBock, V., Mets, T., Romagnoli, M., and Derde, M.P. 1994. Captopril treatment of chronic heart failure in the very old. *J Gerontol* 49: M148-M152.

20. O'Keeffe, S.T., Lye, M., Donnnellan, C., and Carmichael, D.N. 1998. Reproducibility and responsiveness of quality of life assessment and six minute walk test in elderly heart failure patients. *Heart* 80: 377-382.

21. Bernstein, M.L., Despars, J.A., Singh, N.P., Avalos, K., Stansbury, D.W., and Light, R.W. 1994. Re-analysis of the 12-minute walk in patients with COPD. *Chest* 105: 163-167.

22. Hajiro, T., Nishimura, K., Tsukino, M., Ikeda, A., Koyama, H., and Izumi, T. 1998. Analysis of clinical methods used to evaluate dyspnea in patients with COPD. *Am J Respir Crit Care Med* 158: 1185-1189.

23. Gulmans, V.A.M., vanVeldhoven, N.H.M.J., deMeer, K., and Helders, P.J.M. 1996. The six-minute walking test in children with cystic fibrosis: Reliability and validity. *Pediatr Pulmonol* 22: 85-89.

24. Nixon, P.A., Joswiak, M.L., and Fricker, F.J. 1996. A six-minute walk test for assessing exercise tolerance in severely ill children. *J Pediatr* 129: 362-366.

25. Bittner, V. 1997. Six-minute walk test in patients with cardiac dysfunction. *Cardiologia* 42: 897-902.

26. Peeters, P., and Mets, T. 1996. The 6-minute walk as an appropriate exercise test in elderly patients with chronic heart failure. *J Gerontol* 51A: M147-M151.

27. Zugck, C., Kruger, C., Durr, S., Gerber, S.H., Haunstetter, A., Hornig, K., Kubler, W., and Haass, M. 2000. Is the 6-minute walk test a reliable substitute for peak oxygen uptake in patients with dilated cardiomyopathy? *Eur Heart J* 21: 540-549.

28. Montgomery, P.S., and Gardner, A.W. 1998. The clinical utility of a six-minute walk test in peripheral arterial occlusive disease patients. *J Am Geriatr Soc* 46: 706-711.

29. Cahan, M.A., Montgomery, P., Otis, R.B., Clancy, R., Flinn, W., and Gardner, A. 1999. The effect of cigarette smoking status on six-minute walk distance in patients with intermittent claudication. *Angiology* 50: 537-546.

30. King, S., Wessel, I., Bhambhani, Y., Maikala, R., Sholter, D., and Maksymowych, W. 1999. Validity and reliability of the 6-minute walk in persons with fibromyalgia. *J Rheumatol* 26: 2233-2237.

31. Enright, P.L., McBurnie, M.A., Bittner, V., Tracy, R.P., McNamara, R., and Newman, A.B. The Cardiovascular Health Study. The six-minute walk test: A quick measure of functional status in elderly adults. *Chest* (In press).

32. Bittner, V., Weiner, D.H., Yusuf, S., Rogers, W.I., McIntyre, K.M., Bangdiwala, S.I., Kronenberg, M.W., Kostis, J.B., Kohn, R.M., Guillotte, M., et al. 1993. Prediction of mortality and morbidity with a 6-minute walk test in patients with left ventricular dysfunction. *JAMA* 270: 1702-1707.

33. Cahalin, L.P., Mathier, M.A., Semigran, M.J., Dec, G.W., and DiSalvo, T.G. 1996. The six-minute walk test predicts peak oxygen uptake and survival in patients with advanced heart failure. *Chest* 110: 325-332.

34. Cote, C.G., and Celli, B.R. 1998. In patients with COPD, the 6-minute walking distance is a better predictor of health care utilization than FEV_1, blood gases, and dyspnea [abstract]. *Eur Respir J* 383.

35. Kessler, R., Faller, M., Fourgaut, G., Mennecier, B., and Weitzenblum, E. 1999. Predictive factors of hospitalization for acute exacerbation in a series of 64 patients with chronic obstructive pulmonary disease. *Am J Respir Crit Care Med* 159: 158-164.

36. Cahalin, L., Pappagianopoulos, P., Prevost, S., Wain, J., and Ginns, L. 1995. The relationship of the 6-minute walk test to maximal oxygen consumption in transplant candidates with end-stage lung disease. *Chest* 108: 452-459.

37. Guyatt, G.H., Thompson, P.J., Berman, L.B., Sullivan, M.J., Townsend, M., Jones, N.L., and Pugsley, S.O. 1985. How should we measure function in patients with chronic heart and lung disease? *J Chronic Dis* 38: 517-524.

38. Guyatt, G.H., Townsend, M., Keller, J., Singer, J., and Nogradi, S. 1991. Measuring functional status in chronic lung disease: Conclusions from a random control trial. *Respir Med* 85(Suppl B): 17-21.

39. Niederman, M.S., Clemente, P.H., Fein, A.M., Feinsilver, S.H., Robinson, D.A., Ilowite, J.S., and Bernstein, M.G. 1991. Benefits of a multidisciplinary pulmonary rehabilitation program: Improvements are independent of lung function. *Chest* 99: 798-804.

40. Noseda, A., Carpiaux, J., Prigogine, T., and Schmerber, J. 1989. Lung function, maximum and submaximum exercise testing in COPD patients: Reproducibility over a long interval. *Lung* 167: 247-257.

41. Knox, A.J., Morrison, J.F., and Muers, M.F. 1988. Reproducibility of walking test results in chronic obstructive airways disease. *Thorax* 43: 388-392.

42. Guyatt, G.H., Pugsley, S.O., Sullivan, M.J., Thompson, P.J., Berman, L.B., Jones, N.L., Fallen, E.L., and Taylor, D.W. 1984. Effect of encouragement on walking test performance. *Thorax* 39: 818-822.

43. Leger, L.A. 1982. A maximal multistage 20-m shuttle run test to predict $\dot{V}O_2$ max. *Eur J Appl Physiol* 49: 1-12.

44. Singh, S.J., Morgan, M.D.L., Scott, S., Walters, D., and Hardman, A.E. 1992. Development of a shuttle walking test of disability in patients with chronic airways obstruction. *Thorax* 47: 1019-1024.

45. Revill, S.M., Morgan, M.D.L., Singh, S.J., Williams, J., and Hardman, A.E. 1999. The endurance shuttle walk: A new field test for the assessment of endurance capacity in chronic obstructive pulmonary disease. *Thorax* 54: 213-222.

46. Singh, S.J., Morgan, M.D.L., Hardman, A.E., Rowe, C., and Bardsley, P.A. 1994. Comparison of oxygen uptake during a conventional treadmill test and the

shuttle walking test in chronic airflow limitation. *Eur Respir J* 7: 2016-2020.

47. Morales, F.J., Martinez, A., Mendez, M., Agarrado, A., Ortega, F., Fernandez-Guerra, J., Montemayor, T., and Burgos, J. 1999. A shuttle walk test for assessment of functional capacity in chronic heart failure. *Am Heart J* 138: 292-298.

48. Enright, P.L., and Sherrill, D.L. 1998. Reference equations for the six-minute walk in healthy adults. *Am J Respir Crit Care Med* 158: 1384-1387.

49. Barst, R.J., Rubin, L.J., McGoon, M.D., Caldwell, E.J., Long, W.A., and Levy, P.S. 1994. Survival in primary pulmonary hypertension with long-term continuous intravenous prostacyclin. *Ann Intern Med* 121: 409-415.

50. Miyamoto, S., Nagaya, N., Satoh, T., Kyotani, S., Sakamaki, F., Fujita, M., Nakanishi, N., and Miyatake, K. 2000. Clinical correlates and prognostic significance of six-minute walk test in patients with primary pulmonary hypertension. *Am J Respir Crit Care Med* 161: 487-492.

51. Guyatt, G.H., Sullivan, M.J., Thompson, P.J., Fallen, E.L., Pugsley, S.O., Taylor, D.W., and Berman, L.B. 1985. The 6-minute walk: A new measure of exercise capacity in patients with chronic heart failure. *Can Med Assoc J* 132: 919-923.

52. Lipkin, D.P., Scrivin, A.J., Crake, T., and Poole-Wilson, P.A. 1986. Six-minute walking test for assessing exercise capacity in chronic heart failure. *BMJ* 292: 653-655.

53. Troosters, T., Gosselink, R., and Decramer, M. 1999. Six-minute walking distance in healthy elderly subjects. *Eur Respir J* 14: 270-274.

54. Weiss, R.A., et al. 2000. Six minute walk test in severe COPD: Reliability and effect of walking course layout and length. Paper presented at ACCP Conference; September 2000; San Francisco.

55. Stevens, D., Elpern, E., Sharma, K., Szidon, P., Ankin, M., and Kesten, S. 1999. Comparison of hallway and treadmill six-minute walk tests. *Am J Respir Crit Care Med* 160: 1540-1543.

56. Jensen, L.A., Onyskiw, J.E., and Prasad, N.G.N. 1998. Meta-analysis of arterial oxygen saturation monitoring by pulse oximetry in adults. *Heart Lung* 27: 387-408.

57. Barthelemy, J.C., Geyssant, A., Riffat, J., Antoniadis, A., Berruyer, J., and LaCour, J.R. 1990. Accuracy of pulse oximetry during moderate exercise: A comparative study. *Scand J Clin Lab Invest* 50: 533-539.

58. Borg, G.A. 1982. Psychophysical bases of perceived exertion. *Med Sci Sports Exerc* 14: 377-381.

59. Leach, R.M., Davidson, A.C., Chinn, S., Twort, C.H.C., Cameron, I.R., and Batemen, N.T. 1992. Portable liquid oxygen and exercise ability in severe respiratory disability. *Thorax* 47: 781-789.

60. Mungall, I.P.F., and Hainsworth, R. 1979. Assessment of respiratory function in patients with chronic obstructive airways disease. *Thorax* 34: 254-258.

61. Roberts, C.M., Bell, J., and Wedzicha, J.A. 1996. Comparison of the efficacy of a demand oxygen delivery system with continuous low flow oxygen in subjects with stable COPD and severe oxygen desaturation on walking. *Thorax* 51: 831-834.

62. Hay, J.G., Stone, P., Carter, J., Church, S., Eyre-Brook, A., Pearson, M.G., Woodcock, A.A., and Calverley, P.M. 1992. Bronchodilator reversibility, exercise performance and breathlessness in stable chronic obstructive pulmonary disease. *Eur Respir J* 5: 659-664.

63. Grove, A., Lipworth, B.J., Reid, P., Smith, R.P., Lamage, L., Ingram, C.G., Jenkins, R.J., Winter, J.H., and Dhillon, D.P. 1996. Effects of regular salmeterol on lung function and exercise capacity in patients with COPD. *Thorax* 51: 689-693.

64. Redelmeier, D.A., Bayoumi, A.M., Goldstein, R.S., and Guyatt, G.H. 1997. Interpreting small differences in functional status: The six-minute walk test in chronic lung disease patients. *Am J Respir Crit Care Med* 155: 1278-1282.

65. Weiner, P., Magadle, R., Berar-Yanay, N., Davidovich, A., and Weiner, M. 2000. The cumulative effect of long-acting bronchodilators, exercise, and inspiratory muscle training on the perception of dyspnea in patients with advanced COPD. *Chest* 118: 672-678.

66. Bittner, V., Sanderson, B., Breland, J., Adams, C., and Schuman, C. 2000. Assessing functional capacity as an outcome in cardiac rehabilitation: Role of the 6 minute walk test. *Clin Exerc Physiol.*

index

Note: Information contained in tables or figures are indicated by an italicized *t* or *f*.

about the AACVPR

Founded in 1985, the American Association of Cardiovascular and Pulmonary Rehabilitation (AACVPR) is dedicated to the professional development of its members through information, networking, and educational opportunities. Central to the mission is the improvement in the quality of life for patients and their families.

Guiding Principles

- Quality and integrity are never compromised.

- Customers are the focus of everything we do.

- Creating and maintaining constancy of purpose is an ongoing responsibility.

- Stewardship and creative risk taking are compatible.

- Creating and cultivating productive partnerships and alliances help position AACVPR in an ever-changing health care industry.

- Creating and maintaining a learning environment helps maintain our freshness and keeps us on the cutting edge.

- Continuous improvement is essential to our success.

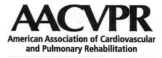

American Association of
Cardiovascular and Pulmonary Rehabilitation
Membership Application

Name_____

Professional Degree _____
(Please list no more than two)

Title_____

Place of Employment_____

Mailing Address_____

City_____

State/Province_____

Zip Code/Postal Code _____

Country _____

This address is: ❑ Home ❑ Business

(The above address will be used for mailings and will be listed in the Membership Directory.)

Email:_____

(Be sure to include your email address for frequent Regulatory Updates and the monthly News and Views. The AACVPR does not distribute email addresses to other groups).

Daytime Phone: (   )_____

Fax: (   ) _____

Are you a current member of your state/regional society?

❑ Yes ❑ No

General Information

Where did you hear about the AACVPR?

❑ From an AACVPR Member

❑ Was a Previous Member—Year(s)

❑ Journal of Cardiopulmonary Rehabilitation

❑ Professional Colleague

❑ State/Regional Society

❑ University/School

❑ Other

What made you decide to join the AACVPR? _____

_____

Membership Categories

❑ Member
Membership Fee $150
Shall be any interested person of majority age who is a nurse, physician, medical scientist, allied health-care practitioner or educator, and who in his or her professional endeavors, is regularly involved in some aspect of cardiovascular and/or pulmonary rehabilitation. Members have AACVPR voting privileges.

Which of these categories best represents you?
Check only one:
❑ Behavioral Scientist
❑ Cardiopulmonary Physical Therapist
❑ Exercise Rehabilitation Specialist
❑ Cardiovascular Physician
❑ Exercise Physiologist
❑ Pulmonary Physician
❑ Nutritionist/Dietician
❑ Pulmonary Nurse
❑ Respiratory Therapist
❑ Cardiovascular Nurse
❑ Other _____

Are you certified by a professional association?
❑ Yes ❑ No

Association Name _____

Certification _____

Does your current employer support individual AACVPR membership?
❑ Yes ❑ No

❑ Student Member
Membership Fee $75

A Student Member shall be any interested undergraduate or graduate college student currently carrying the equivalent of at least one half of a full-time academic load for one year, as defined by the university or college of attendance. The area of study must be in a medical or allied health curriculum. Student Membership also applies to physicians-in-training, including residents and interns.

To qualify as a Student Member, one must submit a copy of his or her current student identification card along with this completed application.

Educational Institution _____

Major _____

Year Degree Expected_____

❑ Associate Member
Membership Fee $150

Shall be any person with an interest in cardiovascular and /or pulmonary rehabilitation, but not currently eligible for classification as a Member or Student Member. Dues are established by the Board of Directors and may be changed at its discretion. Associate Member privileges include a subscription to the AACVPR newsletter and placement on the Association mailing list.

Primary Occupation_____

Place of Employment_____

Current Program Involvement

In what area(s) do you spend the majority of your practice?

What is the emphasis of your clinical practice?

Check one:

❑ In-patient Cardiovascular/Pulmonary/Vascular
❑ Out-patient Cardiovascular/Pulmonary/Vascular
❑ In-patient & Out-patient Cardiovascular/Pulmonary/Vascular

Who is your employer?

❑ Hospital   ❑ Educational Institution
❑ Physician/Group practice   ❑ Other: _____

How many new out-patients would you estimate are seen in your program annually?

❑ Less than 100   ❑ 101-200 patients
❑ 201-300 patients   ❑ Over 300 patients

How many new in-patients would you estimate are seen in your program annually?

❑ Less than 100   ❑ 101-500 patients
❑ 501-1000 patients   ❑ Over 1000 patients
❑ Does not apply

Which of the following best describes the emphasis of your work environment?

❑ 100% rehabilitation
❑ 75% rehabilitation/25% prevention
❑ 50% rehabilitation/50% prevention
❑ 25% rehabilitation/75% prevention

Membership Agreement

I certify that the above information is correct and I agree to abide by the Code of Ethical and Professional conduct of the American Association of Cardiovascular and Pulmonary Rehabilitation. Visit the AACVPR Web site for the code of ethics.

Signature _____ Date _____

Payment

Purchase orders are not accepted.
Payment must accompany application.

❑ Check (Payable to AACVPR; US Funds Only)

❑ MC/Visa/American Express—Exp. Date _____

Cardholder's Name _____

Card Number_____

Cardholder's City/State _____

Cardholder's Signature _____

Heart and Lung Foundation Contribution Opportunities

The Heart and Lung Foundation strives to assist the AACVPR in becoming the recognized leader in professional and public education for the field of cardiopulmonary rehabilitation through:

• **Education**
• **Service/Outreach**
• **Research**

All donations are tax deductible.

Yes, I want to do my part to advance my profession by pl__ ing the following:

❑ $25 .... Foundation Supporter
❑ $50 .... Foundation Member
❑ $100 .... Foundation Partner
❑ $250 .... Foundation Sponsor
❑ $500 .... Foundation Patron
❑ $1,000 .... Foundation Benefactor

Foundation benefactors will be acknowledged on the AACVPR Web site.

AACVPR membership is effective July through June 30. Membership is not pro-rated; however, members joining after march 1 will be deferred until July 1. Membership dues are non-refundable, nor deductible as a charitable contribution. Membership dues may be deductible as an ordinary and necessary business expense. Consult your tax advisor for information.

Please send completed application to:

AACVPR National Office

401 N Michigan Avenue, Suite 2200

Chicago, IL 60611

Telephone: 312-321-5146

Email: aacvpr@sba.com

Web site: www.aacvpr.org

Credit Card Users may fax application to:

312-245-1085